THE CLASSIC PUMPKIN COOKBOOK

The Classic Pumpkin Cookbook: Heritage Recipes, from Perfect Pies to Savory Soups

Cover and book designer: Hilary Harkness
Editor: Emily Beaumont
Proofreader: Jenna Barron

Image credits
All images used under license from Shutterstock.com:

Cover: **keebikadidut:** gingham check pattern; **kichikimi:** pumpkin pie, pumpkins and leaves, and soup bowl; **Vera Serg:** fork, knife, and spoon; **Vectorfair:** back cover label.

Interior: **Atriu Photo Gallery**: 123; **Hut_Design:** 57, 93; **injala:** 17; **keebikadidut:** gingham check pattern (throughout); **kichikimi:** 9, 23, 37, 49, 75, 103, 112; **Olga Selyutina:** 29; **Vera Serg:** 2, 32, 39, 108, 131; **Victoria Sergeeva:** 31; **Vectorfair:** chapter label and scrollwork (throughout).

Library of Congress Cataloging-in-Publication Data

Names: Beaumont, Emily editor
Title: The classic pumpkin cookbook/editor: Emily Beaumont.
Description: Cambridge, Minnesota : Adventure Publications, An imprint of AdventureKEEN, [2026] | Includes index. | Summary: "Discover 100 delicious, sweet, and savory recipes that bring the rich flavor of pumpkin to every meal—from cozy breakfasts and hearty dinners to irresistible baked treats and desserts. Pumpkin is one of the most versatile ingredients in the kitchen. While it's often associated with autumn traditions, this flavorful winter squash can be used year-round in everything from soups and dinners to baked goods and desserts. The Classic Pumpkin Cookbook gathers 100 tried-and-true recipes from AdventureKEEN's trusted cookbook collection, featuring fantastic dishes created by 11 authors. These carefully selected recipes highlight the many ways pumpkin can shine in everyday cooking, as well as special occasions"—Provided by publisher.
Identifiers: LCCN 2026016823 (print) | LCCN 2026016824 (ebook) | ISBN 9781647557010 paperback | ISBN 9781647557027 ebook
Subjects: LCSH: Cooking (Pumpkin) | LCGFT: Cookbooks
Classification: LCC TX803.P93 C537 2026 (print) | LCC TX803.P93 (ebook) | DDC 641.6/562--dc23/eng/20260416
LC record available at https://lccn.loc.gov/2026016823
LC ebook record available at https://lccn.loc.gov/2026016824

10 9 8 7 6 5 4 3 2 1

Published by Adventure Publications
An imprint of AdventureKEEN
310 Garfield Street South
Cambridge, Minnesota 55008
(800) 678-7006
adventurepublications.net

Printed in the United States

THE CLASSIC PUMPKIN COOKBOOK

Heritage Recipes, from Perfect Pies to Savory Soups

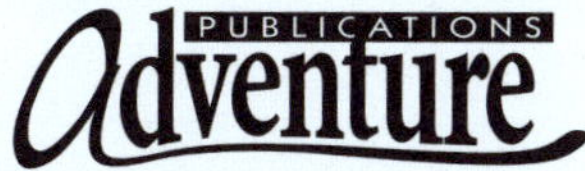

"I'm so glad I live in a world where there are Octobers."

—Lucy Maud Montgomery, *Anne of Green Gables*

PUMPKINS, the symbol of the fall harvest—of Halloween and family and comforts of home and crisp air and woodsmoke—are big round sources of good food and fond memories. One of the most enjoyable experiences of childhood is visiting a local farm, taking a hayride to a pumpkin patch, and selecting the perfect specimen for carving your jack-o'-lantern. But there's so much more you can make with this vibrant winter squash. And, luckily, there are many brands of canned pumpkin available at grocery stores, so you can enjoy the flavor year-round.

As the editor of this cookbook, I've had the pleasure of compiling this collection of 100 recipes, gathered from previously published titles in our catalog. You could say I've gone to the AdventureKEEN garden of recipes and picked these beauties right out of the cookbook patch—planted carefully by 9 authors across 11 titles—and then made them ready for you.

Of course, the first treat that comes to mind is pie. Rest assured, this collection has more than a dozen ideas for that! Importantly, this cookbook also contains recipes for breads, pancakes, muffins, appetizers, side dishes, stews, cakes, cookies, and ice-cream desserts. If you're so inspired, you could even have a whole day of pumpkin meals: Try Julia's Pumpkin Waffles for breakfast, Creamy Pumpkin Soup for lunch, Toasted Pumpkin Seeds as an afternoon snack, Turkey-and-Winter Squash Pot Pie for dinner, and Frosted Pumpkin Cupcakes for dessert! No matter what you decide to make with pumpkins, you'll create new cozy memories in the kitchen with these classic recipes from AdventureKEEN.

—*Emily*

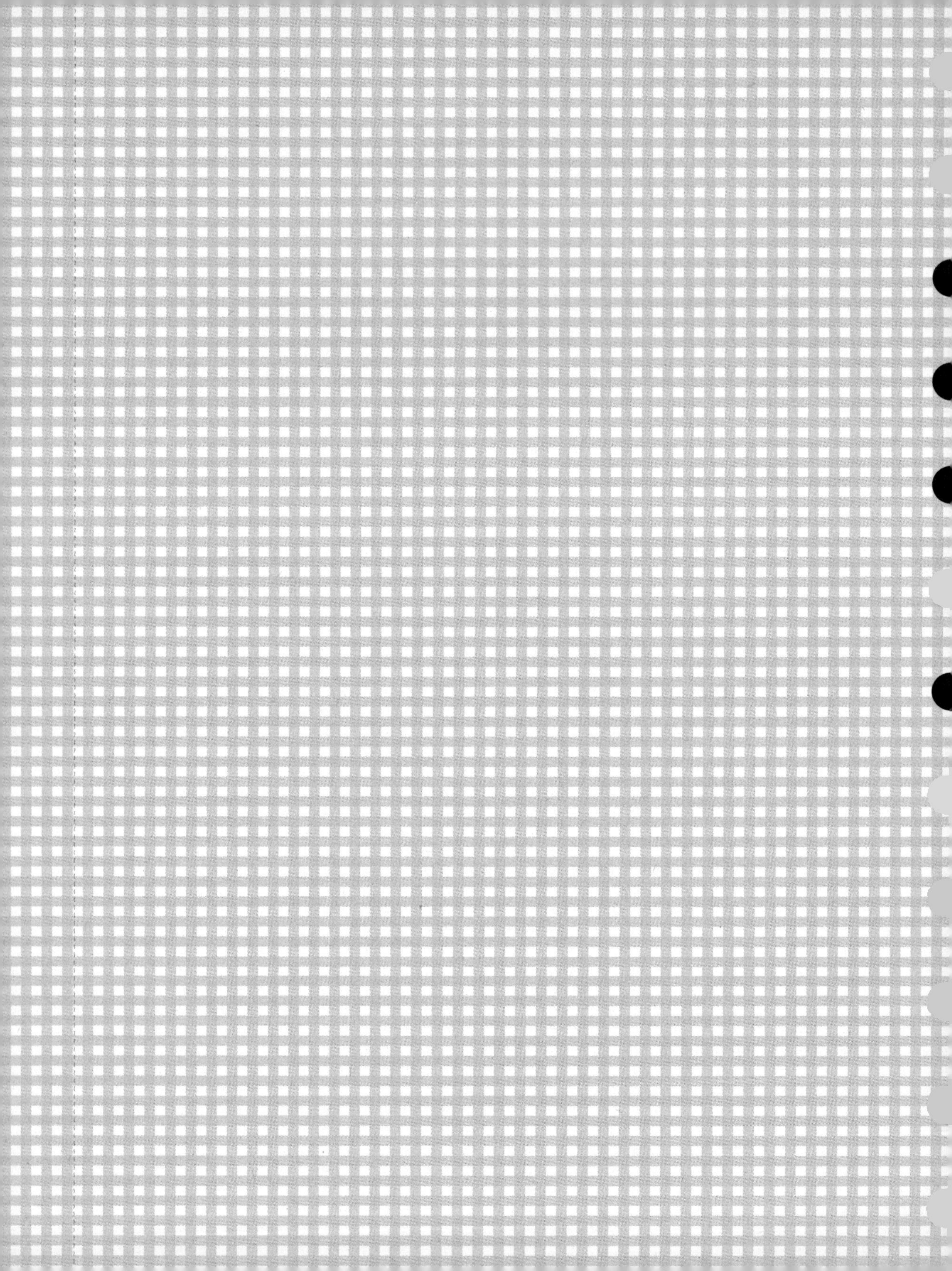

Table of Contents

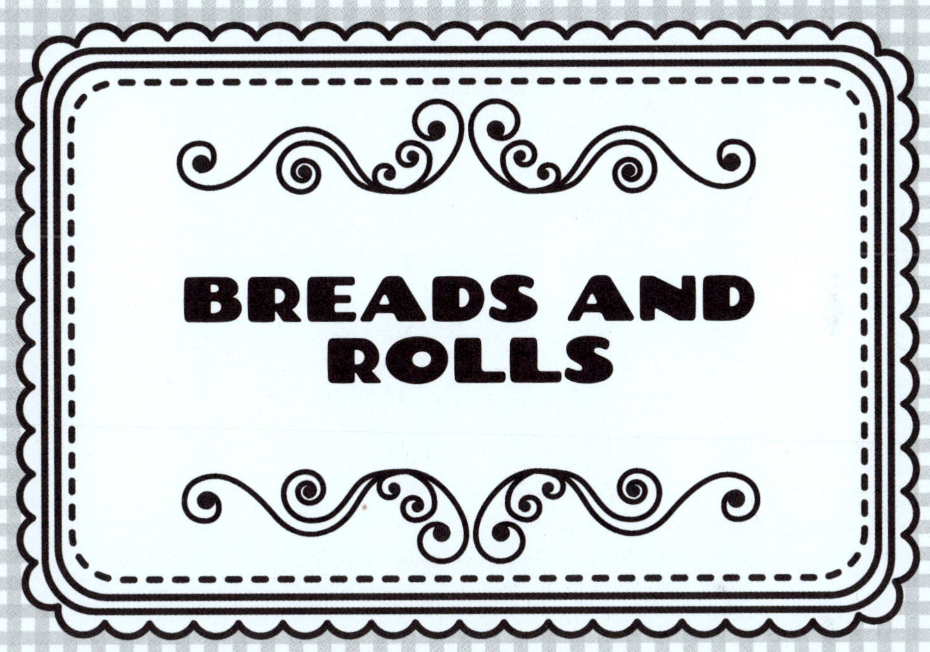

BREADS AND ROLLS

Pumpkin Cornbread

Makes 2 loaves

---

1. Preheat oven to 350°. Combine cornmeal, flour, sugar, baking powder, and baking soda in a large bowl. In a separate large bowl, beat together eggs, oil, pumpkin, and milk. Add pumpkin mixture to cornmeal mixture, gently folding in with a rubber spatula, until batter is smooth and fluffy.

2. Pour batter into 2 loaf pans or 1 (9x13-inch) baking pan. Place on middle rack of oven and bake for 25 minutes or until a wooden pick inserted in center comes out clean. Let cool for 10 minutes before slicing and serving.

2 cups cornmeal

2 cups all-purpose flour

1 cup granulated sugar

2 tablespoons baking powder

½ teaspoon baking soda

4 eggs

1 cup vegetable oil

2¼ cups pumpkin puree

1 cup milk

Notes

Recipe from Holly Harden, *Recipes for Gatherings from Mrs. Sundberg's Kitchen*

Banana-Winter Squash Quick Bread

Makes 2 loaves

Vegetable cooking spray

3 cups all-purpose flour

2 cups granulated sugar

2 teaspoons baking soda

1½ teaspoons baking powder

1½ teaspoons ground cinnamon

1 teaspoon salt

¼ teaspoon ground ginger

¼ teaspoon ground cloves

3 eggs

1 cup vegetable oil

2 teaspoons vanilla extract

1 cup cooked butternut squash or pumpkin

1 cup mashed ripe bananas

1 cup chopped walnuts or pecans

1. Preheat oven to 350°. Lightly grease 2 (8x4-inch) loaf pans with cooking spray.

2. Combine flour, sugar, baking soda, baking powder, cinnamon, salt, ginger, and cloves in a large bowl.

3. In a separate bowl, beat eggs; stir in oil, vanilla, squash, and bananas. Add squash mixture to flour mixture, stirring just until moistened. Fold in chopped walnuts. Pour batter equally into prepared pans.

4. Bake for 1 hour or until a wooden pick inserted in center comes out clean. Cool in pans for 10 minutes. Remove from pans; cool on a wire rack. Refrigerate leftovers.

Notes

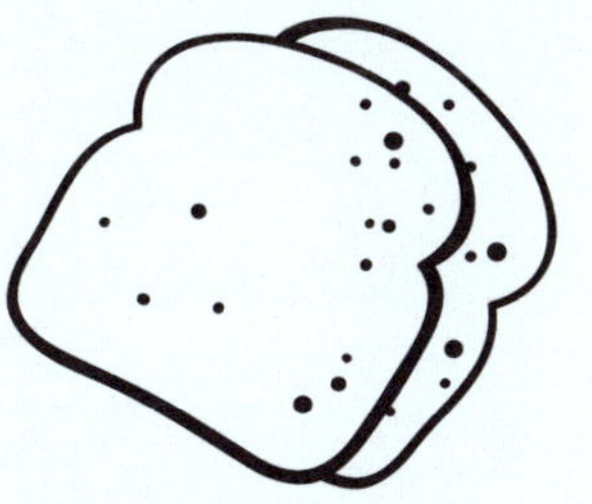

Recipe from Theresa Millang, *The Joy of Squash*

Pumpkin Bread

Makes 2 loaves

Vegetable cooking spray

3½ cups all-purpose flour

2 teaspoons baking soda

1½ teaspoons salt

1 teaspoon ground cinnamon

1 teaspoon ground nutmeg

2 cups granulated sugar

1 cup vegetable oil

4 large eggs

⅔ cup milk or water

1 (15-ounce) can pumpkin (not pie mix)

1 cup chocolate chips (optional)

1. Preheat oven to 350°. Line 2 (9x5-inch) loaf pans with aluminum foil and grease with cooking spray (or use nonstick aluminum foil).

2. Combine flour, baking soda, salt, cinnamon, and nutmeg in a large bowl.

3. In a separate bowl, beat together sugar, oil, eggs, milk, and pumpkin. Stir in chocolate chips, if desired. Stir pumpkin mixture into flour mixture. Spoon batter into prepared pans.

4. Bake for 1 hour or until a wooden pick inserted in center comes out clean.

5. Cool in pans on a wire rack for 10 minutes. Remove from pans and cool completely.

Notes

Recipe from Julia Rutland, *Squash: 50 Tried & True Recipes*

Chocolate Chip Pumpkin Bread

Makes 2 loaves

4 cups all-purpose flour

2 teaspoons baking soda

1 teaspoon salt

1 teaspoon ground cinnamon

½ teaspoon ground nutmeg

2 cups granulated sugar

¾ cup butter, softened

4 eggs

1 (15-ounce) can pumpkin (not pie mix)

1 teaspoon vanilla extract

½ cup cold water

1 cup semisweet mini-chocolate chips

¼ cup chopped pecans

1. Preheat oven to 350°. Grease (with butter) and flour bottoms of 2 (8x4-inch) loaf pans.

2. Combine flour, baking soda, salt, cinnamon, and nutmeg in a large bowl.

3. In the bowl of a stand-up electric mixer, beat sugar and butter on medium speed until creamy. Beat in eggs. Reduce speed to low. Beat in pumpkin, vanilla, and ½ cup water. Add flour mixture, a little at a time, beating until just moistened. Stir in chocolate chips and pecans. Spread batter into prepared pans.

4. Bake for 65 to 75 minutes or until a wooden pick inserted in center comes out clean. Cool in pans for 10 minutes. Remove from pans; cool on a wire rack. Refrigerate leftovers.

Notes

____

____

____

____

____

Recipe from Theresa Millang, *The Joy of Squash*

Favorite Pumpkin-Pecan Bread

Makes 32 servings

½ cup butter

1 (8-ounce) package cream cheese, softened

2½ cups granulated sugar

4 eggs

1 (15-ounce) can pumpkin (not pie mix)

1 teaspoon vanilla extract

3½ cups all-purpose flour

2 teaspoons baking soda

½ teaspoon baking powder

1 teaspoon salt

1 teaspoon ground cinnamon

¼ teaspoon ground cloves

⅛ teaspoon ground ginger

1 cup coarsely chopped pecans

1. Preheat oven to 350°. Grease (with butter) and flour 2 (9x5-inch) loaf pans.

2. In the bowl of a stand-up mixer, beat butter, cream cheese, and sugar on medium speed until creamy. Beat in eggs, 1 at a time. Add pumpkin and vanilla; beat on low speed just until blended.

3. In a separate large bowl, combine flour, baking soda, baking powder, salt, cinnamon, cloves, and ginger. Add flour mixture to pumpkin mixture, a little at a time, beating on low speed until blended. Stir in pecans by hand. Pour batter equally into prepared pans.

4. Bake for 55 to 60 minutes or until a wooden pick inserted in center comes out clean. Cool completely on a wire rack before serving. Store in the refrigerator.

Notes

Recipe from Theresa Millang, *The Joy of Squash*

Pumpkin-Carrot-Raisin Bread

Makes 2 loaves

- Vegetable cooking spray
- 3 cups all-purpose flour
- 2 teaspoons baking soda
- 5 teaspoons pumpkin pie spice
- 1½ teaspoons salt
- 3 cups granulated sugar
- 1 (15-ounce) can pumpkin (not pie mix)
- 4 eggs
- 1 cup vegetable oil
- ½ cup water
- 1 teaspoon vanilla extract
- 1 cup shredded carrots
- 1 cup raisins

1. Preheat oven to 350°. Lightly grease (with cooking spray) and flour 2 (9x5-inch) loaf pans.

2. Combine flour, baking soda, pie spice, and salt in a large bowl.

3. In the bowl of a stand-up mixer, beat sugar, pumpkin, eggs, oil, ½ cup water, and vanilla on medium speed until just blended. Add pumpkin mixture to flour mixture, stirring just enough to moisten.

4. Stir in carrots and raisins. Spoon batter equally into prepared pans.

5. Bake for 60 to 65 minutes or until a wooden pick inserted in center comes out clean. Cool in pans on a wire rack for 10 minutes. Remove from pans, and cool on a wire rack. Store in the refrigerator.

Notes

Recipe from Theresa Millang, *The Joy of Squash*

Oatmeal-Pumpkin Bread

Makes 1 loaf

1 cup quick oats

1 cup milk, heated

¾ cup canned pumpkin (not pie mix)

2 eggs, beaten

¼ cup butter, melted and cooled

1 teaspoon vanilla extract (optional)

2 cups all-purpose flour

1 cup granulated sugar

1 tablespoon baking powder

1 teaspoon ground cinnamon

¼ teaspoon ground nutmeg

⅛ teaspoon ground cloves

¼ teaspoon salt

1 cup raisins

½ cup chopped pecans

1. Preheat oven to 350°. Grease (with butter) a 9x5-inch loaf pan.

2. Mix oats and milk together in a large bowl; let stand for 5 minutes. Stir in pumpkin; eggs; butter; and, if desired, vanilla.

3. In a separate large bowl, combine flour, sugar, baking powder, cinnamon, nutmeg, cloves, and salt; gradually add flour mixture to oat mixture, stirring to combine.

4. Stir in raisins and pecans. Spread batter into prepared pan.

5. Bake for 55 to 60 minutes or until a wooden pick inserted in center comes out clean. Cool in pan for 5 minutes. Remove from pan; cool on a wire rack. Refrigerate leftovers.

Recipe from Theresa Millang, *The Joy of Squash*

Pumpkin Seed Breadsticks

Makes 24 breadsticks

Vegetable cooking spray

All-purpose flour

1 (14-ounce) package refrigerated pizza dough

1 egg, lightly beaten

3 tablespoons shelled pumpkin seeds

Coarse salt

1. Preheat oven to 425°. Lightly grease 2 large baking sheets with cooking spray.

2. Unroll pizza dough onto a lightly floured surface. Using hands, shape dough into a 12x9-inch rectangle. Brush dough with egg. Sprinkle with seeds and salt. Using a floured pizza cutter, slice dough crosswise into ½-inch-wide strips. Place strips onto prepared baking sheets.

3. Bake, 1 sheet at a time, for 8 to 10 minutes or until golden brown. Remove from pan; cool on a wire rack. Refrigerate leftovers.

Notes

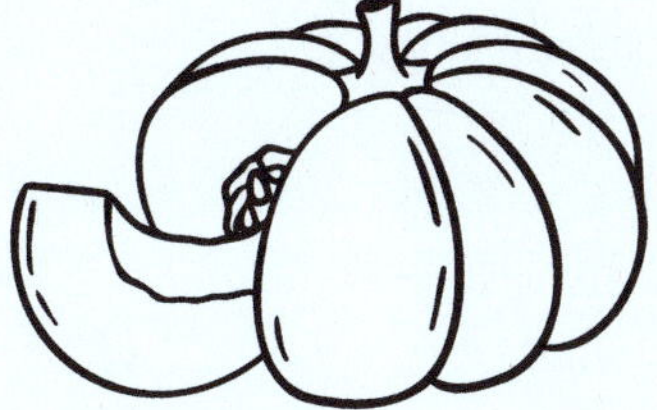

Recipe from Theresa Millang, *The Joy of Squash*

Pumpkin-and-Pepita Parker House Rolls

Makes 1½ dozen

---

7 tablespoons butter, at room temperature and divided

½ cup pumpkin or butternut squash puree

1 cup heavy cream, half-and-half, or whole milk, at room temperature

2 large eggs, at room temperature and divided

¼ cup granulated sugar

3½ cups all-purpose flour

1 envelope (2½ teaspoons) active dry yeast

1½ teaspoons salt

Vegetable oil

Pepitas (roasted pumpkin seeds)

Flaky sea salt

1. Melt 4 tablespoons butter. Pour into the bowl of a stand-up electric mixer. Add pumpkin, cream, 1 egg, sugar, flour, yeast, and salt; mix until a dough forms. Knead on a lightly floured surface (or in mixing bowl with a dough hook) for about 5 minutes or until smooth. Transfer to a lightly oiled bowl, turning to coat surface. Cover loosely with plastic wrap and let rise in a warm place (85°), free from drafts, for 1 to 2 hours or until doubled in bulk.

2. Melt remaining 3 tablespoons butter. Brush a 9x9-inch baking dish lightly with some of the melted butter. Set aside.

3. Punch dough down and divide into 18 pieces on a floured surface. Roll into balls and place in prepared baking dish. Brush tops with remaining melted butter. Cover with plastic wrap and let rise in a warm place for 45 minutes or until puffed (but not doubled in size).

4. Preheat oven to 350°. Whisk remaining egg and brush over tops of rolls. Sprinkle with pepitas and sea salt. Bake for 20 to 25 minutes or until golden brown.

Notes

____

____

____

____

____

Recipe from Julia Rutland, *Squash: 50 Tried & True Recipes*

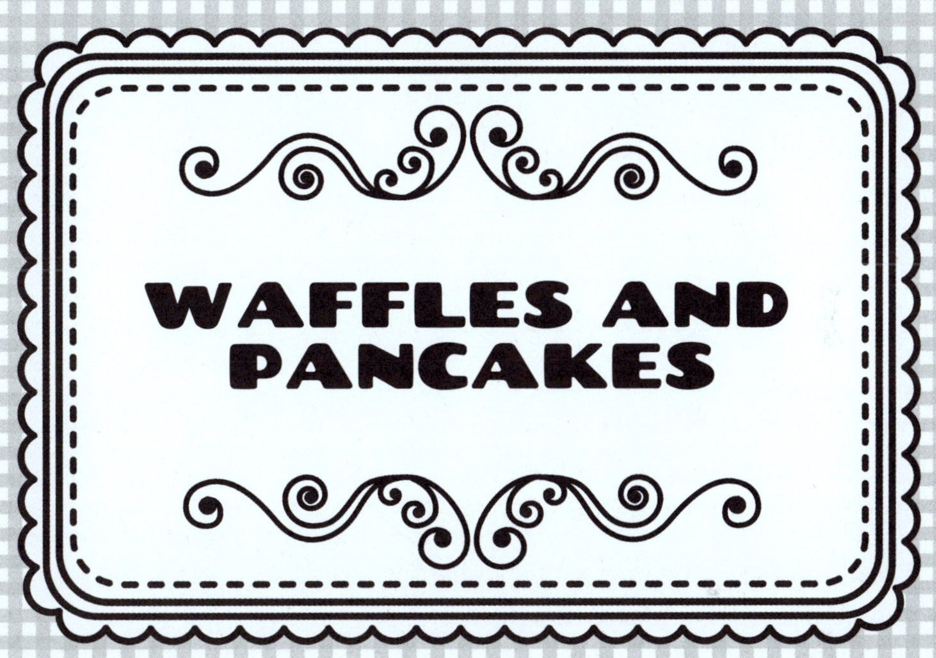

WAFFLES AND PANCAKES

Corrine's Pumpkin Waffles

Makes 6 waffles

2 cups all-purpose flour

⅓ cup granulated sugar

2 teaspoons baking powder

½ teaspoon salt

½ teaspoon ground cinnamon

¼ teaspoon ground ginger

⅛ teaspoon freshly ground nutmeg

6 tablespoons unsalted butter, cubed and chilled

½ cup whole milk

½ cup heavy cream

⅓ cup pumpkin puree

3 eggs

1 teaspoon vanilla or maple extract

Vegetable cooking spray

Toppings: sour cream, softened butter, warm maple syrup, pepitas (roasted pumpkin seeds)

1. Preheat waffle iron.

2. In the bowl of a food processor with a metal blade, pulse flour, sugar, baking powder, salt, cinnamon, ginger, and nutmeg to combine. Sprinkle cold butter pieces on top and process until mixture forms coarse crumbs. Transfer to a large bowl; make a well in center of mixture.

3. In a large glass measuring cup, whisk milk, cream, pumpkin, eggs, and vanilla to combine. Pour milk mixture into well of flour mixture and gently combine. (A few lumps are desired.)

4. Lightly grease waffle iron with cooking spray; cook according to manufacturer's instructions. (It usually takes about ½ cup batter per waffle.) Keep waffles crisp in a low-temperature oven until ready to serve. If necessary, reheat waffles on buttered waffle iron for 30 seconds. Serve waffles hot with desired toppings.

Recipe from Corrine Kozlak, *Maple Syrup: 40 Tried & True Recipes*

Julia's Pumpkin Waffles

Makes 8 waffles

1. Preheat waffle iron.

2. Combine flour, baking powder, baking soda, ground cinnamon, salt, ginger, and cloves in a large bowl.

3. In a separate bowl, whisk together eggs, pumpkin, brown sugar, and buttermilk. Add egg mixture to flour mixture, stirring gently until a moist batter forms.

4. Brush waffle iron with oil. For each 4-inch waffle, spoon about ½ cup batter into iron. Cook for 3 to 5 minutes or until cooked through. Serve with maple syrup and sweetened whipped cream.

2 cups all-purpose flour

2 teaspoons baking powder

½ teaspoon baking soda

2 teaspoons ground cinnamon

1 teaspoon salt

½ teaspoon ground ginger

¼ teaspoon ground cloves

3 large eggs

1 (15-ounce) can pumpkin (not pie mix)

½ cup light brown sugar, firmly packed

1½ cups buttermilk or milk

3 tablespoons vegetable oil or cooking spray

Maple syrup

Sweetened whipped cream

Notes

____

____

____

Recipe from Julia Rutland, *Squash: 50 Tried & True Recipes*

Theresa's Pumpkin Waffles

Makes 8 waffles

½ cup plus 2 tablespoons butter, softened and divided

1 cup plus 2 tablespoons all-purpose flour

½ teaspoon baking powder

½ teaspoon salt

¼ teaspoon baking soda

1 teaspoon ground cinnamon

⅛ teaspoon ground nutmeg

2 tablespoons light brown sugar, firmly packed

1 cup whole milk

½ cup canned pumpkin (not pie mix)

2 eggs, lightly beaten

¼ cup toasted chopped pecans

1 tablespoon orange marmalade

Vegetable cooking spray

1. Preheat waffle iron. Melt 2 tablespoons butter and set aside.

2. Combine flour, baking powder, salt, baking soda, cinnamon, nutmeg, and brown sugar in a large bowl.

3. In a separate bowl, whisk together milk, pumpkin, eggs, and reserved melted butter. Add pumpkin mixture to flour mixture, stirring until just combined. (Do not overmix.)

4. Stir together remaining ½ cup butter, pecans, and marmalade.

5. Lightly grease waffle iron with cooking spray; cook according to manufacturer's instructions. (It usually takes about ½ cup batter per waffle). Serve waffles warm with butter mixture. Refrigerate leftovers.

Recipe from Theresa Millang, *The Joy of Squash*

Pumpkin Pancakes

Makes 6 servings

1½ cups buttermilk

1 cup canned pumpkin (not pie mix)

1 egg

2 tablespoons vegetable oil

2 cups all-purpose flour

3 tablespoons light brown sugar, firmly packed

2 teaspoons baking powder

1 teaspoon baking soda

1 teaspoon ground cinnamon

½ teaspoon salt

½ teaspoon ground ginger

¼ teaspoon ground cloves

1. Lightly grease a pancake griddle or skillet with vegetable oil. Preheat griddle.

2. Combine buttermilk, pumpkin, egg, and oil in a large bowl.

3. In a separate bowl, combine flour, brown sugar, baking powder, baking soda, cinnamon, salt, ginger, and cloves. Stir flour mixture into pumpkin mixture just until combined. (Do not overmix.)

4. For each pancake, pour ¼ cup batter onto griddle; cook until brown on both sides. Serve warm. Refrigerate leftovers.

Notes

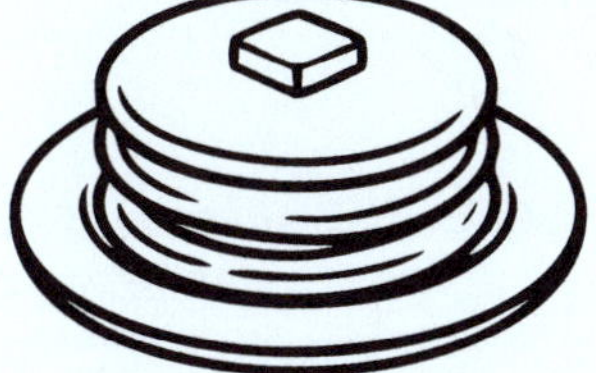

Recipe from Theresa Millang, *The Joy of Squash*

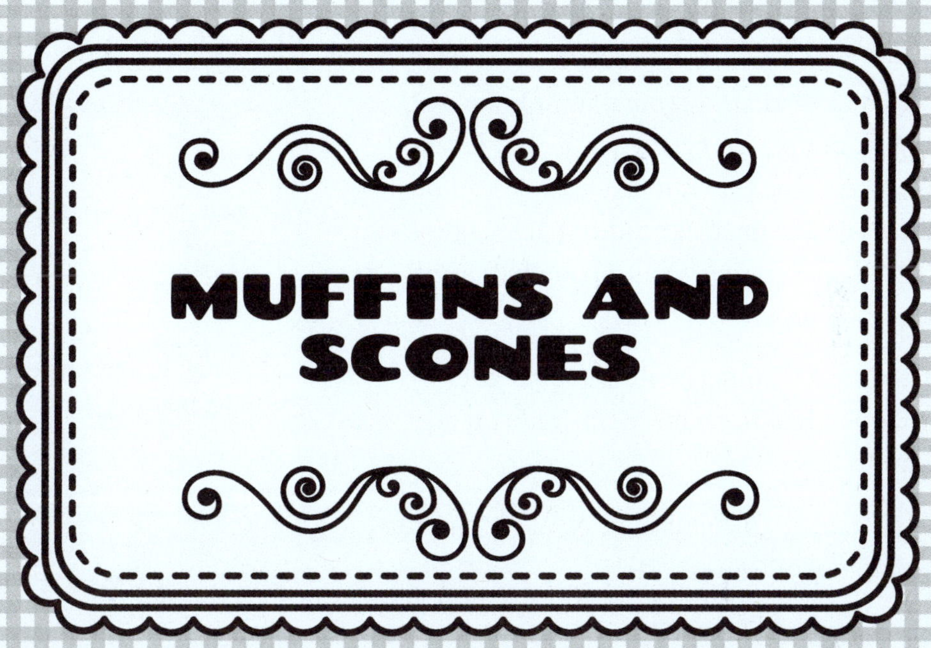

MUFFINS AND SCONES

Pumpkin-Raisin Muffins

Makes 30 muffins

---

1 (30-ounce) can pumpkin pie mix

2 (15.4-ounce) packages nut quick bread and muffin mix (such as Pillsbury)

1 egg, lightly beaten

1 cup raisins

Vegetable cooking spray

2 tablespoons granulated sugar

1 teaspoon ground cinnamon

1. Preheat oven to 375°.

2. To make batter, combine pumpkin pie mix, nut bread mix, and egg in a large bowl. Mix just until bread mix is moistened. Stir in raisins. Place cupcake liners in muffin pans; lightly grease with cooking spray. Spoon batter into prepared cups, filling ¾ full.

3. To make topping, combine sugar and cinnamon in a small bowl. Sprinkle on top of muffins.

4. Bake for 15 to 20 minutes or until tops are golden brown.

Notes

Recipe from Margie Knoblauch and Mary Brubacher, *North Country Cabin Cooking*

Maple-Frosted Pumpkin Muffins

Makes 10 muffins

Vegetable cooking spray

1 cup whole-wheat flour

¾ cup all-purpose flour

1 teaspoon baking soda

½ teaspoon baking powder

½ teaspoon ground cloves

½ teaspoon ground cinnamon

½ teaspoon ground nutmeg

¼ teaspoon salt

6 tablespoons granulated sugar

1 cup pumpkin puree

¼ cup vegetable oil

¼ cup maple syrup

1½ tablespoons milk

2 eggs

Maple Glaze (recipe at left)

Garnish: toasted pumpkin seeds

1. Preheat oven to 350°. Lightly grease muffin pans with cooking spray.

2. Combine flours, baking soda, baking powder, cloves, cinnamon, nutmeg, salt, and sugar in a large bowl. Make a well in center of mixture.

3. In a large glass measuring cup, beat together pumpkin, oil, ¼ cup maple syrup, milk, and eggs. Pour pumpkin mixture into well of flour mixture and gently combine. Scoop batter into prepared muffin pans, filling ¾ full. Bake for 20 minutes or until a toothpick inserted in center comes out clean. Cool. Drizzle with Maple Glaze and garnish, if desired.

Maple Glaze: Melt **3 tablespoons butter** in a saucepan over medium heat; whisk in **⅓ cup maple syrup.** Bring to a boil and cook, stirring constantly, for 2 minutes. Remove from heat and stir in **¼ teaspoon maple extract.** Sift in **¾ cup powdered sugar** and whisk until smooth and slightly thick.

Recipe from Corrine Kozlak, *Maple Syrup: 40 Tried & True Recipes*

Pumpkin-Cream Cheese Streusel Muffins

Makes 24 muffins

- 1 (8-ounce) package cream cheese, softened
- 2½ cups granulated sugar, divided
- 1 teaspoon vanilla extract
- 4 eggs, divided
- 3⅓ cups all-purpose flour, divided
- 4 teaspoons ground cinnamon, divided
- 4 tablespoons butter
- ⅓ cup chopped pecans
- 1 teaspoon ground cloves
- ½ teaspoon ground nutmeg
- ½ teaspoon ground ginger
- 1 teaspoon baking soda
- 1 teaspoon salt
- 1 (15-ounce) can pumpkin (not pie mix) or butternut squash
- 1 cup vegetable oil

1. Preheat oven to 375°. Place 24 cupcake liners in 2 (12-cup) muffin pans.

2. Combine cream cheese, ½ cup sugar, vanilla, and 1 egg in a small bowl; set aside.

3. Combine another ½ cup sugar, ⅓ cup flour, and 1 teaspoon cinnamon in a small bowl; cut in butter with a pastry blender or fork until large crumbs form. Stir in pecans. Set aside.

4. Combine remaining 3 cups flour, remaining 3 teaspoons cinnamon, cloves, nutmeg, ginger, baking soda, and salt in a large bowl.

5. Whisk together remaining 3 eggs, remaining 1½ cups sugar, pumpkin, and oil in a large bowl. Add pumpkin mixture to flour mixture, stirring just until moistened. Spoon half of batter into prepared muffin pans. Dollop cream cheese mixture evenly over batter in pans, and top evenly with remaining batter. Sprinkle with reserved pecan mixture.

6. Bake for 20 minutes. Remove from pan; cool on a wire rack.

Recipe from Julia Rutland, *Squash: 50 Tried & True Recipes*

Chocolate Chip Pumpkin Muffins

Makes 36 muffins

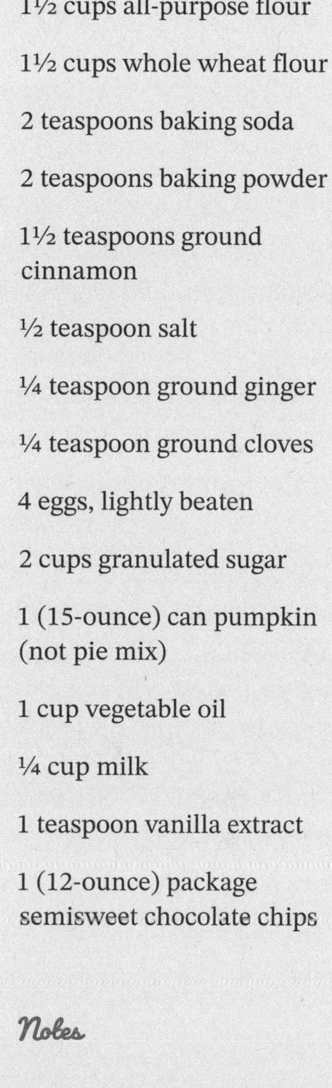

1½ cups all-purpose flour

1½ cups whole wheat flour

2 teaspoons baking soda

2 teaspoons baking powder

1½ teaspoons ground cinnamon

½ teaspoon salt

¼ teaspoon ground ginger

¼ teaspoon ground cloves

4 eggs, lightly beaten

2 cups granulated sugar

1 (15-ounce) can pumpkin (not pie mix)

1 cup vegetable oil

¼ cup milk

1 teaspoon vanilla extract

1 (12-ounce) package semisweet chocolate chips

Notes

____

____

____

1. Preheat oven to 400°. Place 36 cupcake liners in 3 (12-cup) muffin pans.

2. Combine flours, baking soda, baking powder, cinnamon, salt, ginger, and cloves in a large mixing bowl.

3. In a separate bowl, combine eggs, sugar, pumpkin, oil, milk, and vanilla, stirring until blended. Add pumpkin mixture to flour mixture, stirring just enough to moisten. Stir in chocolate chips. Spoon batter equally into prepared muffin pans.

4. Bake for 20 to 25 minutes or until tops spring back when touched. Cool in pans for 5 minutes. Remove from pans; cool on a wire rack. Refrigerate leftovers.

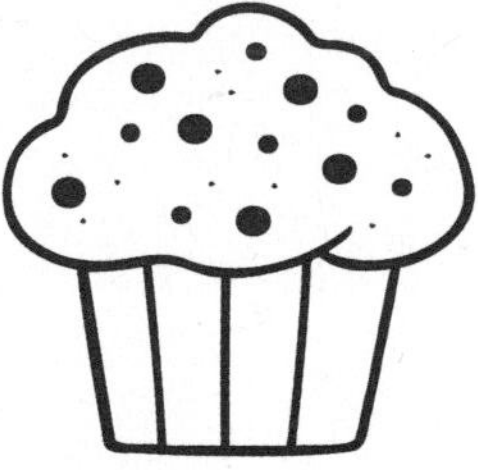

Recipe from Theresa Millang, *The Joy of Squash*

Pumpkin Scones

Makes 12 scones

---

1. Preheat oven to 375°.

2. To make dough, beat butter and brown sugar in a large bowl on medium speed until creamy. Add pumpkin, milk, egg yolk, and ½ teaspoon vanilla; beat until blended.

3. In a separate bowl, mix together flour, baking powder, cinnamon, salt, ginger, and cloves. Stir flour mixture into butter mixture. Stir in raisins. Drop dough by rounded ¼-cupfuls onto an ungreased baking sheet. Bake for 20 to 25 minutes or until edges are lightly browned and scones are set. Remove from baking sheet. Cool on a wire rack.

4. To make glaze, whisk together powdered sugar, remaining ½ teaspoon vanilla, and 1 tablespoon orange juice in a small bowl (adding more juice, if necessary, to reach desired consistency). Drizzle glaze over baked scones. Refrigerate leftovers.

½ cup butter, softened

½ cup light brown sugar, firmly packed

1 cup canned pumpkin (not pie mix)

¼ cup whole milk

1 egg yolk

1 teaspoon vanilla extract, divided

2½ cups all-purpose flour

2 teaspoons baking powder

1 teaspoon ground cinnamon

½ teaspoon salt

½ teaspoon ground ginger

½ teaspoon ground cloves

½ cup golden raisins

1 cup powdered sugar

1 to 2 tablespoons orange juice

Notes

Recipe from Theresa Millang, *The Joy of Squash*

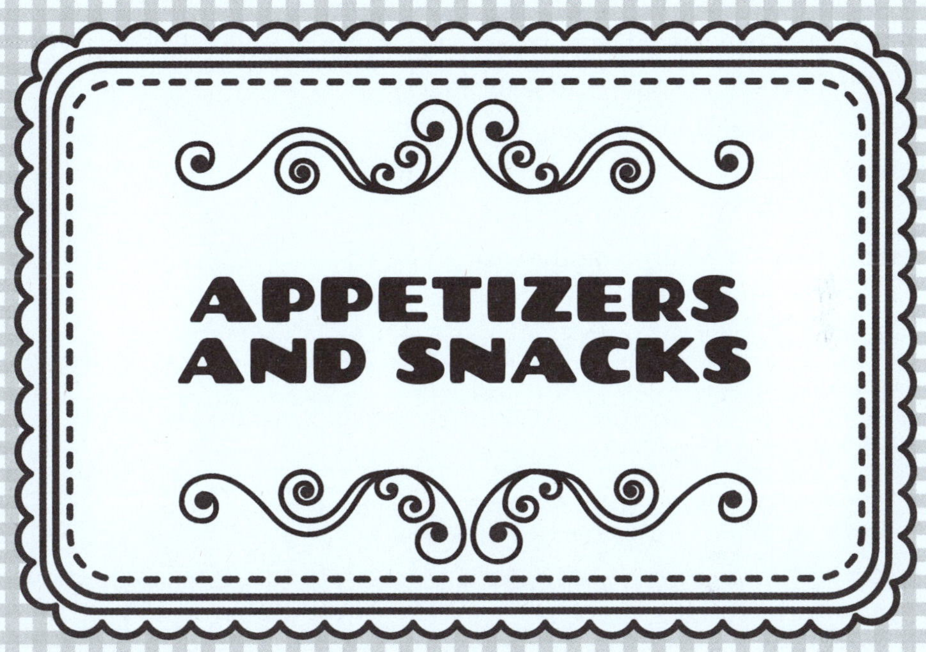

APPETIZERS AND SNACKS

Toasted Pumpkin Seeds

2 cups fresh pumpkin seeds

2 tablespoons vegetable oil

Salt, garlic salt, or seasoned salt to taste

1. Preheat oven to 250°.

2. Place seeds in a bowl of cold water, and clean pumpkin fibers from seeds with your fingers. Rinse seeds in a colander and dry completely on paper towels. Spread seeds out on a baking sheet. Sprinkle with oil. Sprinkle generously with salt. Bake for 30 to 45 minutes, stirring occasionally, until light golden brown. Transfer to paper towels to cool; store toasted seeds in an airtight container.

Notes

Recipe from Teresa Marrone, *The Seasonal Cabin Cookbook*

Spicy Pumpkin Seeds

Makes 4 servings

Vegetable cooking spray

2 cups fresh pumpkin seeds

1 tablespoon butter, melted

1 teaspoon Worcestershire sauce

1 teaspoon granulated sugar

½ teaspoon salt

¼ teaspoon garlic powder

⅛ teaspoon ground red pepper

1. Preheat oven to 250°.

2. Line a rimmed baking sheet with aluminum foil; lightly grease foil with cooking spray.

3. Mix together seeds, butter, Worcestershire sauce, sugar, salt, garlic powder, and red pepper in a bowl, stirring gently to coat. Spread seed mixture out on prepared baking sheet. Bake, stirring often, for about 1 hour or until seeds are dry and lightly browned. Remove from oven. Cool completely. Store in an airtight container.

Notes

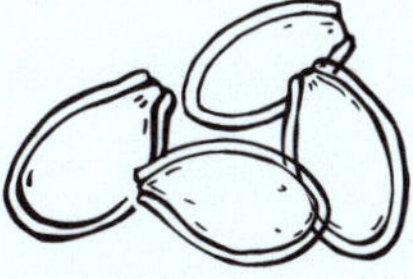

Recipe from Theresa Millang, *The Joy of Squash*

Pumpkin Hummus

Makes 3 cups

---

1 (15-ounce) can pumpkin (not pie mix)

1 (15-ounce) can garbanzo beans, rinsed and drained

½ teaspoon grated lemon zest

⅓ cup fresh lemon juice

⅓ cup tahini

1 garlic clove, sliced

2 tablespoons extra-virgin olive oil

1½ teaspoons ground cumin

1 teaspoon salt

¼ teaspoon smoked paprika or ground cayenne pepper

Garnish: toasted pumpkin seeds

Pita chips

1. Combine pumpkin, beans, lemon zest and juice, tahini, garlic, oil, cumin, salt, and paprika in a food processor; process until smooth.

2. Spoon into a serving bowl; garnish, if desired. Serve with pita chips.

Notes

____

____

____

____

Recipe from Julia Rutland, *Squash: 50 Tried & True Recipes*

Pumpkin Dip

Makes 3 cups

1 (8-ounce) package cream cheese, softened

2 cups pumpkin pie mix

2 cups powdered sugar

1 teaspoon ground cinnamon

¼ to ½ teaspoon ground ginger

Gingersnaps

1. Beat cream cheese in a large bowl until smooth. Beat in pumpkin pie filling. Add powdered sugar, cinnamon, and ginger; mix well. Serve with gingersnaps. Store in refrigerator.

Notes

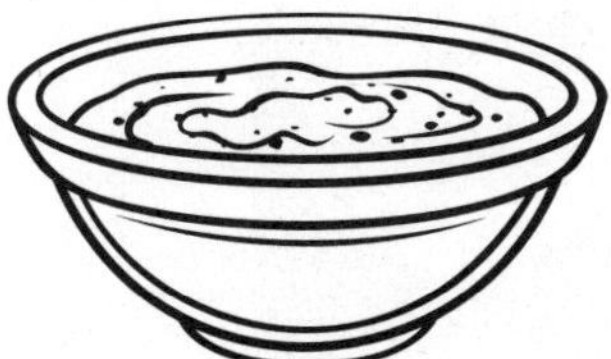

Recipe from Holly Harden, *Recipes for Gatherings from Mrs. Sundberg's Kitchen*

Quick Pumpkin Butter

Makes 1¼ cups

1 cup canned pumpkin (not pie mix)

½ cup honey

¼ cup molasses

1 tablespoon lemon juice

¾ teaspoon ground cinnamon

⅛ teaspoon ground cloves

1. Combine pumpkin, honey, molasses, lemon juice, cinnamon, and cloves in a saucepan. Bring mixture to a boil, stirring often. Reduce heat. Simmer, uncovered, for about 15 minutes or until thickened. Spoon into a clean glass container. Chill for 1 hour before serving. Store in the refrigerator.

Notes

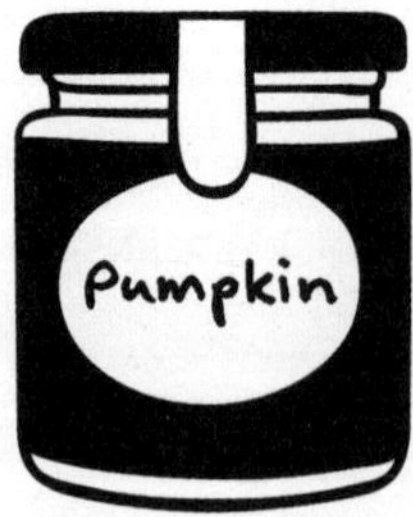

Recipe from Theresa Millang, *The Joy of Squash*

Winter Squash-and-Quinoa Salad Cups

Makes 4 to 6 servings

---

5 cups diced butternut squash or pumpkin

2 tablespoons extra-virgin olive oil

1 teaspoon salt

1 cup plain or tricolor quinoa

2 cups vegetable or chicken broth

½ cup dried cranberries

⅓ cup toasted pepitas (roasted pumpkin seeds) or walnuts

⅓ cup chopped red onion

Honey-Thyme Vinaigrette (recipe at left)

1. Preheat oven to 400º.

2. Toss squash with 2 tablespoons oil in a large bowl; sprinkle with 1 teaspoon salt. Spread squash out on a baking sheet. Bake for 15 to 20 minutes or until tender.

3. Place quinoa in a wire-mesh sieve and rinse under running water. Bring broth to a boil in a medium-size saucepan. Stir in quinoa. Cover and cook for 15 to 20 minutes or until tender and broth is mostly absorbed. Let stand, covered, for 5 minutes. (Drain if any liquid pools at bottom of pan.) Fluff with a fork.

4. Combine squash, quinoa, cranberries, pepitas, and onion in a large bowl. Drizzle with Honey-Thyme Vinaigrette, tossing to combine. Serve in 4 to 6 individual cups.

Honey-Thyme Vinaigrette: Whisk together **¼ cup apple cider vinegar; 1 teaspoon Dijon mustard; 1 tablespoon honey; 1 small garlic clove, minced; 2 teaspoons chopped fresh thyme; ½ teaspoon salt; ¼ teaspoon coarsely ground black pepper;** and **⅓ cup extra-virgin olive oil** in a bowl until well blended. Makes about ¾ cup.

Notes

Recipe from Julia Rutland, *Squash: 50 Tried & True Recipes*

SIDE DISHES

Roasted Winter Squash-and-Pomegranate Salad

Makes 6 servings

4 to 4½ cups cubed butternut squash or pumpkin

2 tablespoons extra-virgin olive oil

½ teaspoon salt

¼ teaspoon coarsely ground black pepper

3 cups baby spinach

3 cups baby arugula

½ cup pomegranate seeds

1 (8-ounce) container burrata or fresh mozzarella, cut into pieces

Pecan Vinaigrette (recipe at left)

1. Preheat oven to 350°.

2. Place squash in a bowl. Add 2 tablespoons oil, ½ teaspoon salt, and pepper; toss to coat. Place in a single layer on a baking sheet. Roast for 20 minutes or until squash is tender but still holds it shape.

3. Combine spinach and arugula on a serving platter or individual plates. Top evenly with squash, pomegranate seeds, and cheese. Drizzle with Pecan Vinaigrette.

Pecan Vinaigrette: Whisk together **¼ cup Champagne or white wine vinegar, 2 tablespoons maple syrup, 1 minced shallot, 1 teaspoon Dijon mustard,** and **½ teaspoon salt.** Slowly whisk in **½ cup extra-virgin olive oil.** Whisk in **½ cup toasted-and-chopped pecan halves.** Makes 1 cup.

Notes

Recipe from Julia Rutland, *Squash: 50 Tried & True Recipes*

Roasted Sugar Pumpkin

Makes 3 cups

1 (3-pound) sugar pumpkin

1. Preheat oven to 375°.

2. Place whole pumpkin onto a baking sheet. Using a skewer, poke through top of pumpkin several times to vent steam while baking. Bake for about 1 hour or until fork-tender. Remove pumpkin from oven; let cool for 30 minutes.

3. Cut pumpkin in half; discard seeds. Scrape cooked flesh from skin and place in a bowl. Mash until smooth. If not using right away, cover and refrigerate for up to 2 days.

Notes

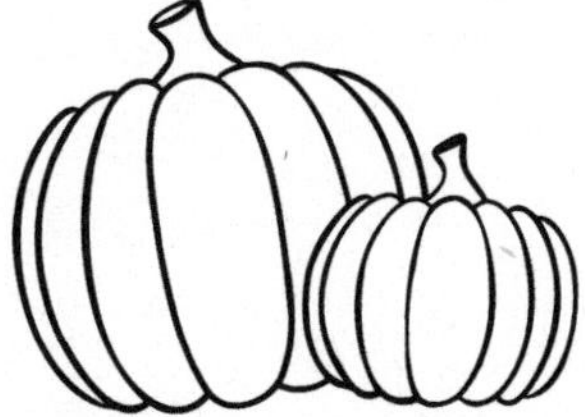

Recipe from Theresa Millang, *The Joy of Squash*

Stuffed Mini-Pumpkins

Makes 4 servings

½ cup uncooked wild rice

3 to 4 cups cold water

4 fresh mini-pumpkins

1 teaspoon fresh orange zest

Juice of 1 large fresh orange

2 tablespoons honey

½ teaspoon salt

¼ teaspoon coarsely ground black pepper

¼ cup dried cranberries

2 tablespoons chopped pecans, toasted

1 teaspoon chopped fresh mint

1. Preheat oven to 375°.

2. Place wild rice in a small saucepan. Cover with 3 to 4 cups water. Bring to a boil over medium-high heat; reduce heat to low and simmer for about 40 minutes or until done (when grains start to pop). Pour cooked rice into a colander and rinse with cold water; drain. Place drained rice in a large bowl.

3. Meanwhile, cut tops off of pumpkins. Scoop out seeds and strings. Place pumpkins, cut-side down, in a baking pan with ½ inch water. Bake for 15 minutes. Remove from oven. Turn pumpkins upright; return to oven and bake for about 10 minutes or until fork-tender. Remove pumpkins to a large platter.

4. Stir together orange zest and juice, honey, salt, pepper, cranberries, pecans, and mint in a small bowl; add to rice and mix well. Stuff rice mixture into cooked pumpkins. Serve warm. Refrigerate leftovers.

Notes

Recipe from Theresa Millang, *The Joy of Squash*

Mashed Pumpkin and Squash

Makes 4 servings

1 small pie pumpkin, peeled, seeded, and cut into small pieces

Yellow squash, peeled, seeded, and cut into small pieces

Maple sugar to taste

1. Place pumpkin and squash pieces into a large pot. Add water to cover. Stir in maple sugar. Cook over low heat until soft enough to mash.

Notes

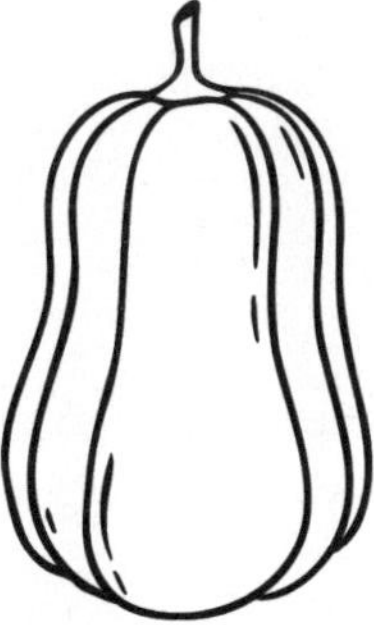

Recipe from Dr. Duane R. Lund, *Cooking Minnesotan You-Betcha!*

Winter Squash Gratin

Makes 6 servings

1 (2-pound) butternut squash or pumpkin

¼ cup butter

3 cloves garlic, finely chopped

¼ teaspoon salt

¼ teaspoon coarsely ground black pepper

¼ teaspoon dried oregano

¼ cup coarse, plain breadcrumbs or panko

¼ cup grated Parmesan cheese

1. Preheat oven to 375°. Lightly grease a 13x9-inch glass baking dish with butter.

2. Peel squash, then cut in half lengthwise; discard seeds. Cut into ½-inch-thick slices. Place slices, overlapping slightly, in prepared baking dish.

3. Melt butter in a small saucepan over low heat. Add garlic; cook and stir for 3 minutes. Set aside 1 tablespoon butter mixture. Brush squash slices with remaining butter mixture. Sprinkle with salt, pepper, and oregano.

4. Stir together breadcrumbs, Parmesan cheese, and 1 tablespoon reserved butter mixture in a bowl; sprinkle evenly over squash. Bake for about 1 hour or until squash is tender and slightly browned.

Notes

Recipe from Theresa Millang, *The Joy of Squash*

Winter Gruyère Gratin

Makes 8 to 10 servings

Butter

1 (3-pound) butternut squash or pumpkin

2 shallots, chopped

2 cups (8 ounces) shredded Gruyère cheese, divided

2 cups heavy cream

1 teaspoon Dijon mustard

2 teaspoons chopped fresh sage

1 teaspoon salt

¾ teaspoon coarsely ground black pepper

Pinch of crushed red pepper flakes

1. Preheat oven to 375°. Lightly grease a 13x9-inch baking dish with butter.

2. Peel squash and cut in half; remove seeds and discard. Cut both squash halves into ⅛-inch slices.

3. Arrange half of squash pieces on bottom of baking dish. Sprinkle with shallots and 1 cup cheese. Top with remaining squash slices and remaining 1 cup cheese.

4. Whisk together cream, mustard, sage, salt, black pepper, and red pepper flakes in a small bowl. Pour over squash slices.

5. Cover with aluminum foil and bake for 1 hour or until squash is tender and almost done. Uncover and bake for 10 to 15 minutes or until golden brown and bubbly.

Notes

Recipe from Julia Rutland, *Squash: 50 Tried & True Recipes*

Winter Squash-and-Onion Tart

Makes 8 servings

3 tablespoons butter, divided

1 large sweet onion, halved and sliced

1 store-bought refrigerated piecrust

2 cups mashed or pureed butternut squash or pumpkin (from about 1 pound cubed)

2 large eggs

½ cup (2 ounces) grated Havarti, Fontina, or gouda cheese

¼ cup shredded Parmesan cheese

2 ounces soft goat cheese, crumbled

1 teaspoon chopped fresh rosemary

½ teaspoon salt

¼ cup panko breadcrumbs

¼ teaspoon coarsely ground black pepper

1. Melt 2 tablespoons butter in a skillet over medium heat. Add onion and cook for 30 to 35 minutes or until golden brown and very tender. Set aside.

2. Preheat oven to 375°. Unfold piecrust and fit into a 9½-inch tart pan with removable bottom. Line bottom with aluminum foil and fill with pie weights, uncooked rice, or dried beans. Bake for 15 minutes. Remove foil and weights; bake for 5 more minutes. Cool.

3. Combine mashed squash, eggs, cheeses, rosemary, and salt in a large bowl. Stir in reserved onion. Spread squash mixture into prepared crust.

4. Melt remaining 1 tablespoon butter in a glass measuring cup. Stir in panko and pepper. Sprinkle over squash. Bake for 40 minutes or until golden brown and set. Cool for 5 minutes before slicing.

Recipe from Julia Rutland, *Squash: 50 Tried & True Recipes*

Louisiana Sweet Potato-Pumpkin Casserole

Makes 18 servings

---

4 pounds sweet potatoes, peeled and cut into 2- to 3-inch pieces

1 (15-ounce) can pumpkin (not pie mix)

½ cup plus ⅓ cup light brown sugar, firmly packed and divided

4 tablespoons butter, softened and divided

½ teaspoon plus ⅛ teaspoon salt, divided

¼ teaspoon coarsely ground black pepper

2 large eggs

1 teaspoon vanilla extract

3 tablespoons all-purpose flour

½ cup chopped pecans

1. Preheat oven to 350°. Grease a 13x9-inch baking dish with butter.

2. Microwave sweet potatoes on a microwave-safe plate for about 15 minutes or until tender. Cool slightly and place in a large bowl. Add pumpkin, ½ cup brown sugar, 3 tablespoons butter, ½ teaspoon salt, and pepper. Mash with a potato masher until lumpy. Add eggs and vanilla; stir until blended. Spoon pumpkin mixture into prepared baking dish.

3. To make topping, combine remaining ⅓ cup brown sugar, flour, remaining 1 tablespoon butter, and remaining ⅛ teaspoon salt in a bowl; sprinkle evenly over pumpkin mixture in baking dish. Sprinkle pecans evenly over top.

4. Bake for about 25 minutes or until thoroughly heated through. Broil for 1 minute or until bubbly and nuts are toasted.

Notes

Recipe from Theresa Millang, *The Joy of Squash*

Winter Squash Holiday Casserole

Makes 8 servings

1 (3-pound) butternut squash or pumpkin (about 3 pounds), peeled, seeded, and cut into small pieces

1 cup whole milk

8 tablespoons butter, melted and divided

3 eggs, lightly beaten

¾ cup granulated sugar

1 teaspoon vanilla extract

1 teaspoon ground cinnamon

⅛ teaspoon ground cloves

⅛ teaspoon ground nutmeg

¼ cup all-purpose flour

½ cup crushed sugar cookies or vanilla wafers

¼ cup light brown sugar, firmly packed

2 tablespoons chopped pecans

1. Preheat oven to 350°. Lightly grease a 2-quart baking dish with butter.

2. Place squash in a large saucepan with enough water to cover. Bring to a boil; reduce heat, cover, and cook for 20 to 30 minutes or until tender. Drain well. Place squash in a large bowl; beat or mash until smooth. Stir in milk, 6 tablespoons melted butter, eggs, granulated sugar, and vanilla until well blended.

3. Combine cinnamon, cloves, nutmeg, and flour in a bowl; stir cinnamon mixture into squash mixture.

4. Spoon mixture into prepared dish. Cover with aluminum foil and bake for 45 minutes. Remove from oven. Remove foil.

5. In a small bowl, mix together cookies, brown sugar, pecans, and remaining 2 tablespoons melted butter; sprinkle evenly over casserole. Return to oven and bake, uncovered, for 10 to 12 minutes or until heated through.

Recipe from Theresa Millang, *The Joy of Squash*

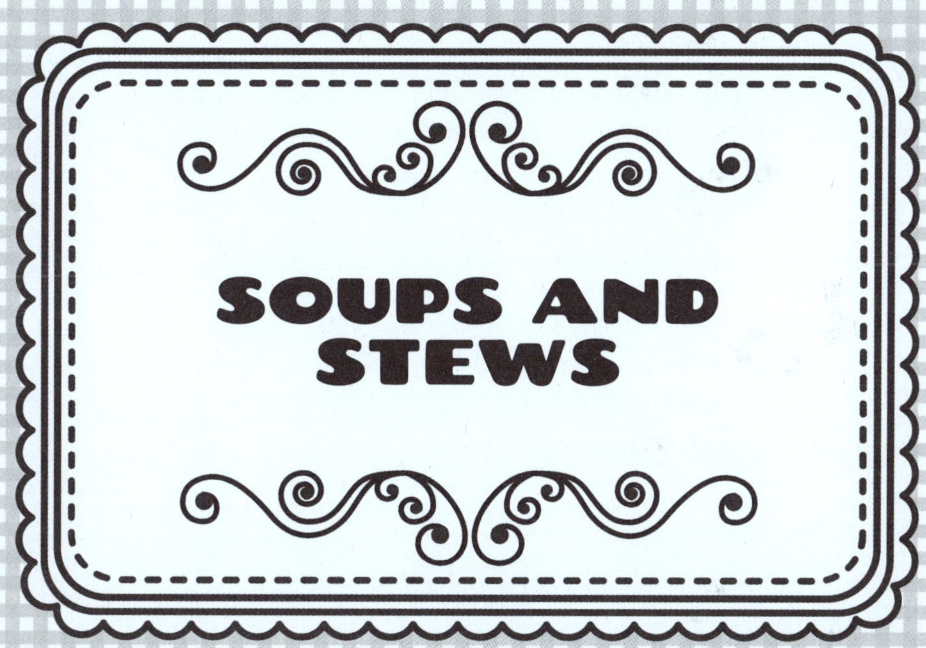

SOUPS AND STEWS

Creamy Pumpkin Soup

Makes 6 servings

1. Melt butter in a large pot. Add onion and garlic; sauté until onion is translucent. Add pumpkin, potatoes, and broth to pot. Bring to a boil; reduce heat and simmer until potatoes are tender. Remove from heat and let cool. Puree pumpkin mixture, in batches, in a blender.

2. Return pumpkin mixture to pot over medium heat. Stir in half-and-half, salt, pepper, and nutmeg. Heat for 20 minutes (do not boil) or until ready to serve. Garnish, if desired.

2 tablespoons butter

1 medium-size onion, chopped

1 clove garlic, minced

2 cups canned or cooked pumpkin

2 cups diced potatoes

2 (14½-ounce) cans chicken broth

2 cups half-and-half

½ teaspoon salt

½ teaspoon coarsely ground black pepper

1 teaspoon ground nutmeg

Garnishes: sour cream, chopped fresh parsley

Notes

Recipe from Dr. Duane R. Lund, *The Soup Cookbook*

Pumpkin Soup

Makes 6 servings

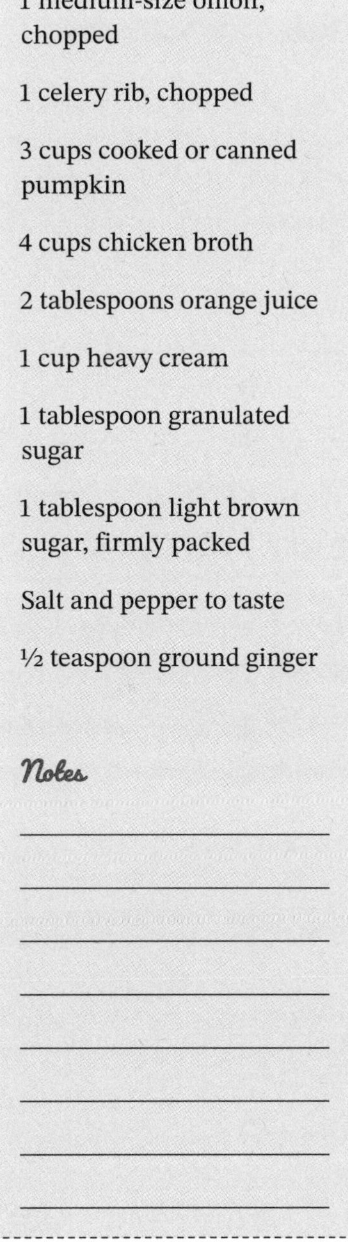

2 tablespoons butter

1 medium-size onion, chopped

1 celery rib, chopped

3 cups cooked or canned pumpkin

4 cups chicken broth

2 tablespoons orange juice

1 cup heavy cream

1 tablespoon granulated sugar

1 tablespoon light brown sugar, firmly packed

Salt and pepper to taste

½ teaspoon ground ginger

Notes

1. Melt butter in a large pot. Add onion and celery; sauté until onion is translucent. Stir in pumpkin, broth, orange juice, cream, sugars, salt, pepper, and ginger. Bring to a boil; reduce heat and simmer for 20 minutes.

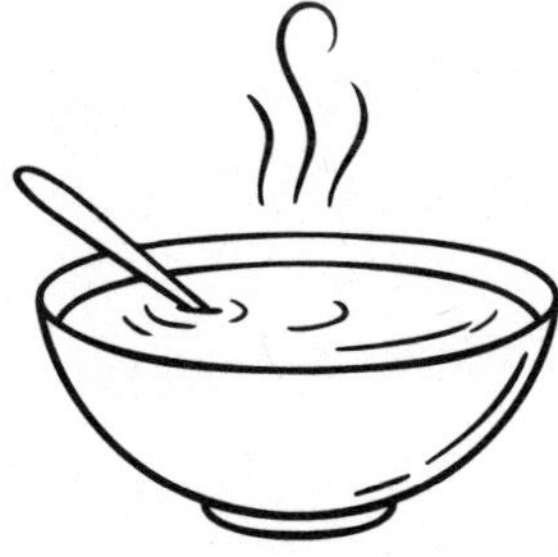

Recipe from Dr. Duane R. Lund, *The Soup Cookbook*

Pumpkin Soup in the Shell

Makes 6 to 8 servings

1 (6- to 8-pound) pumpkin

6 cups chicken broth

1 medium-size onion, chopped

2 apples, peeled and diced

2 carrots, chopped

1 potato, peeled and cubed

8 slices bacon, cooked and crumbled

½ teaspoon rosemary

½ teaspoon basil

1 teaspoon cumin

Garnish: croutons

1. Preheat oven to 350°. Carefully slice pumpkin, removing top ¼ portion of pumpkin. Scoop out seeds and pulp. Replace top. Place pumpkin in a baking dish; bake for 1 hour or until meat is not soft but can be easily scooped. Scoop out meat, leaving a ½-inch shell. Cut meat into bite-size pieces. (Leave oven on.) Return pumpkin shell to baking dish.

2. Pour broth into a large pot over high heat. Stir in onion, apples, carrots, potato, bacon, rosemary, basil, and cumin. Bring soup to a boil; reduce heat and simmer for 30 minutes or until vegetables are tender.

3. Transfer soup to pumpkin shell. Bake for 20 minutes. Garnish, if desired.

Notes

Recipe from Dr. Duane R. Lund, *The Soup Cookbook*

Favorite Pumpkin Soup

Makes 5 servings

- 1/4 cup butter
- 1/3 cup finely chopped onion
- 1/2 cup finely chopped celery
- 1/2 cup finely chopped carrot
- 1 tablespoon minced shallots
- 4 cups canned pumpkin (not pie mix)
- 2 cups chicken broth
- 1 1/2 cups water
- 1/2 cup heavy cream
- 1/4 teaspoon dried thyme
- 1/4 teaspoon coarsely ground black pepper
- Salt to taste
- 1 small French baguette, cut into 1/4-inch slices
- 5 tablespoons blue cheese crumbles

1. Melt butter in a large pot. Add onion, celery, carrot, and shallots; cook over medium heat, stirring constantly, for 3 minutes. Add pumpkin, broth, and 1 1/2 cups water. Cook over medium heat until vegetables are tender. Remove pot from heat.

2. Transfer pumpkin mixture to a food processor or blender; process until smooth. Return to pot. Stir in cream, thyme, pepper, and salt. Heat mixture until warm, but do not boil.

3. Preheat oven to broil. Place bread slices on a baking sheet; broil until crispy. Remove bread from oven; sprinkle with cheese. Serve bread over warm soup.

Recipe from Theresa Millang, *The Joy of Squash*

Curried Pumpkin Soup

Makes 4 servings

2 cups chicken or vegetable broth

1 carrot, diced

Half of 1 (medium-size) onion

1 bay leaf

½ teaspoon crumbled dried thyme

1 (15-ounce) can pumpkin (not pie mix)

½ teaspoon curry powder blend

½ teaspoon salt

⅛ teaspoon coarsely ground black pepper

1 cup heavy cream, half-and-half, or evaporated milk

Garnishes: sour cream, chopped fresh chives

1. In a large pot, combine broth, carrot, onion, bay leaf, and thyme. Bring to a boil; reduce heat and cook for 15 minutes or until vegetables are tender. Remove from heat and allow to cool slightly. Remove and discard bay leaf.

2. Transfer cooled broth mixture to container of a blender; process until smooth. Return broth mixture to pot; add pumpkin, curry, salt, and pepper. Bring just to a boil over medium heat; reduce heat and simmer, stirring occasionally, for 5 to 10 minutes. Stir in cream and cook until heated through. Pour into individual bowls; garnish, if desired.

Notes

____

____

____

____

Recipe from Teresa Marrone, *The Seasonal Cabin Cookbook*

Pumpkin Soup from India

Makes 6 servings

2 medium-size onions, chopped

4 tablespoons vegetable oil

2 tablespoons all-purpose flour

2 cups pumpkin meat, cut into small cubes

5 cups chicken broth

2 cups milk

½ teaspoon curry powder

½ teaspoon ground nutmeg

Salt and pepper to taste

Garnishes: heavy cream, paprika

1. Sauté onion in oil in a large pot until translucent. Add flour, whisking until smooth. Stir in pumpkin, broth, milk, curry, nutmeg, salt, and pepper. Bring to a boil; reduce heat and simmer for 30 minutes or until pumpkin is tender. Remove from heat and let cool.

2. Strain soup mixture through a sieve over a large saucepan; discard pulp. Return soup mixture to pot. Bring to a boil; reduce heat and simmer for 10 minutes or until hot. Garnish, if desired.

Notes

Recipe from Dr. Duane R. Lund, *The Soup Cookbook*

Thai Pumpkin-and-Lentil Soup

Makes 8 cups

1 tablespoon extra-virgin olive oil

½ small onion, finely chopped

2 teaspoons freshly grated ginger

2 garlic cloves, minced

4 cups vegetable or chicken broth

1 (15-ounce) can pumpkin (not pie mix)

1 (13.66-ounce) can coconut milk

1 cup uncooked split red lentils, rinsed

2 tablespoons red curry paste

2 teaspoons lime juice

1½ teaspoons fine sea salt

Garnishes: fresh cilantro, sliced red bell pepper

1. Heat oil in a 5-quart Dutch oven (cocotte) over medium heat. Add onion and cook, stirring frequently, for 3 minutes or until tender. Add ginger and garlic; cook for 1 minute.

2. Stir in broth, pumpkin, coconut milk, lentils, curry paste, lime juice, and salt.

3. Bring mixture to a boil; reduce heat and simmer for 25 minutes or until lentils are tender but still hold their shape. For a smooth soup, puree with an immersion blender. Garnish, if desired.

Notes

____

____

____

Recipe from Julia Rutland, *Cast-Iron Cooking*

Curried Winter Squash Soup

Makes 6 servings

- 2 tablespoons butter
- 6 green onions, finely chopped
- 2 garlic cloves, minced
- 2 green bell peppers, seeded and finely chopped
- ¼ cup minced fresh flat-leaf parsley
- 2 teaspoons minced fresh basil or 1 teaspoon dried basil
- 1 (2-pound) butternut squash or pumpkin, peeled, seeded, and cubed
- 1 (14.5-ounce) can plum tomatoes, undrained
- 4 cups chicken broth
- ½ teaspoon ground allspice
- ¼ teaspoon ground mace
- Pinch of ground nutmeg
- 1 ham bone or ½ pound smoked ham
- 2 teaspoons curry powder
- ¼ teaspoon salt
- ¼ teaspoon coarsely ground black pepper

1. Melt butter in a large pot over medium heat. Add onions, garlic, bell peppers, parsley, and basil. Cook, stirring constantly, for 5 minutes. Stir in squash, tomatoes, broth, allspice, mace, and nutmeg. Add ham bone. Bring to a boil; reduce heat to low and simmer, covered, for 50 to 60 minutes or until squash is tender. Remove and discard ham bone.

2. Strain soup mixture through a sieve into a large saucepan. Place solids in a food processor. Add 1 cup strained liquid to solids in food processor. Puree until smooth.

3. Pour puree back into saucepan. Stir in curry powder. Bring to a boil; reduce heat and simmer for 10 minutes. Stir in salt and pepper. Leftovers may be stored in the refrigerator for up to 3 days.

Recipe from Theresa Millang, *The Joy of Squash*

Spicy Winter Squash Soup

Makes 6 to 8 servings

2 tablespoons extra-virgin olive oil

6 cloves fresh garlic, chopped

2 tablespoons grated ginger

1 jalapeño pepper, seeded and finely chopped

1 tablespoon salt

¼ teaspoon cayenne pepper

4 pounds butternut squash or pumpkin, peeled, seeded, and cut into 2-inch cubes

3 cups chicken broth

1 tablespoon light brown sugar, firmly packed

3 cups cold water

3 tablespoons heavy cream

1. Heat oil in a large pot over high heat. Add garlic, ginger, jalapeño, and salt. Cook, stirring constantly, for 1 minute or until vegetables are tender but not brown. Add cayenne pepper, stirring for 30 seconds.

2. Add squash, broth, brown sugar, and 3 cups water. Bring to a boil. Reduce heat and simmer, stirring occasionally, for 20 minutes or until squash is tender.

3. Puree soup mixture, in batches, in a blender until smooth. Return to pot. Stir in cream just before serving.

Notes

____

Recipe from Theresa Millang, *The Joy of Squash*

Quick Pumpkin Soup with Apple

Makes 4 servings

1 (15-ounce) can pumpkin (not pie mix), pureed if necessary

1 (14½-ounce) can chicken broth

1 cup applesauce

½ teaspoon allspice

1 teaspoon ground cinnamon

Salt and pepper to taste

1. Place pumpkin, broth, applesauce, allspice, and cinnamon in a large pot over medium-high heat. Stir in salt and pepper; cook, stirring occasionally, until heated through.

Notes

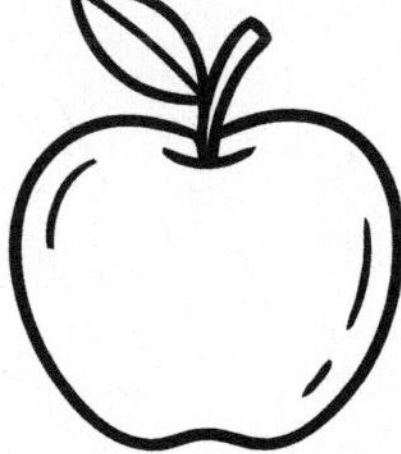

Recipe from Dr. Duane R. Lund, *The Soup Cookbook*

Winter Squash, Kale, and Cannellini Soup

Makes 6 servings

- 2 tablespoons extra-virgin olive oil
- 1 onion, chopped
- 1 stalk celery, chopped
- 6 garlic cloves, minced
- 1 tablespoon Italian seasoning
- 6 cups chicken broth
- 2 large carrots, chopped
- 1 (28-ounce) can diced tomatoes, undrained
- ⅓ cup tomato paste
- 3½ to 4 cups diced butternut squash or pumpkin (about 1¼ to 1½ pounds)
- 6 cups coarsely chopped fresh kale
- 1 (15.5-ounce) can cannellini beans, rinsed and drained
- Salt and pepper to taste

1. Heat oil in a Dutch oven or soup pot over medium-high heat. Add onion, celery, garlic, and Italian seasoning. Cook, stirring often, for 5 minutes or until vegetables are slightly softened.

2. Add broth, carrots, tomatoes, tomato paste, and squash. Bring to a boil; reduce heat and simmer, covered, for 15 to 20 minutes or until vegetables are tender. Stir in kale and beans. Cook for 5 minutes, stirring occasionally, until kale wilts and soup is heated through. Season with salt and pepper.

Recipe from Julia Rutland, *Squash: 50 Tried & True Recipes*

Black Bean-and-Winter Squash Chili

Makes 10 cups

---

3 tablespoons olive oil

1 large onion

2 garlic cloves, minced

2 poblano peppers, chopped

1 red bell pepper, chopped

2 cups vegetable broth

2 (15-ounce) cans black beans, rinsed and drained

1 (28-ounce) can diced fire-roasted or chili seasoned tomatoes, undrained

1 (8-ounce) can tomato sauce

2 tablespoons chili powder

1 tablespoon ground cumin

2 teaspoons smoked paprika

½ teaspoon salt

¼ teaspoon coarsely ground black pepper

3½ to 4 cups cubed or chopped butternut squash or pumpkin

Toppings: sour cream, shredded cheddar cheese, fresh cilantro

1. Heat oil in a large pot over medium heat. Add onion and cook, stirring frequently, for 5 minutes or until tender. Add garlic; cook for 2 minutes. Add poblanos and red bell peppers. Cook for 5 minutes, stirring constantly.

2. Stir in broth, beans, tomatoes, tomato sauce, chili powder, cumin, paprika, salt, and black pepper. Stir in squash. Bring to a boil; reduce heat and cook for 25 minutes or until squash is tender. Serve with desired toppings.

Recipe from Julia Rutland, *Squash: 50 Tried & True Recipes*

Turkey-Pumpkin Chili

Makes 6 servings

2 tablespoons vegetable oil

1 medium-size onion, chopped

1 small green bell pepper, chopped

3 cloves fresh garlic, finely chopped

1 jalapeño pepper, seeded and finely chopped

1 pound ground turkey meat

1 (14-ounce) can diced tomatoes

1 (15-ounce) can pumpkin (not pie mix)

1 cup water

1 tablespoon chili powder

1 teaspoon ground cumin

½ teaspoon dried oregano

¼ teaspoon coarsely ground black pepper

Salt to taste

1 (15-ounce) can kidney beans, drained

1. Heat oil in a large pot over medium-high heat. Add onion, bell pepper, and garlic; cook, stirring often, for about 4 minutes or until vegetables are tender. Stir in jalapeño.

2. Add turkey to pot; cook, stirring often, until browned. Add tomatoes, pumpkin, 1 cup water, chili powder, cumin, oregano, black pepper, and salt. Bring mixture to a boil. Stir in beans. Reduce heat; cover and simmer, stirring occasionally, for 30 minutes.

Recipe from Theresa Millang, *The Joy of Squash*

MAIN DISHES

Honey-Mustard Chicken-and-Squash Sheet Pan Supper

Makes 4 servings

¼ cup plus 1 tablespoon extra-virgin olive oil, divided

¼ cup honey

2 tablespoons whole-grain mustard

2 tablespoons Dijon mustard

2 teaspoons lemon juice

½ teaspoon paprika or smoked paprika

Salt and pepper to taste

4 skin-on, bone-in chicken leg quarters or thighs

2 pounds thin-skinned or peeled butternut squash or pumpkin, cut into large chunks (about 8 cups)

1 large sweet onion, cut into pieces

8 small garlic cloves, peeled

1. Preheat oven to 425°. Line a rimmed baking sheet with aluminum foil (lightly greased with olive oil) or parchment paper.

2. Combine ¼ cup oil, honey, mustards, lemon juice, paprika, salt, and pepper in a bowl. Set aside ¼ cup honey-mustard mixture.

3. Heat remaining 1 tablespoon oil in a heavy skillet over medium-high heat. Add chicken and sear for 3 to 4 minutes on each side.

4. Place chicken on prepared pan and brush with some of the honey-mustard mixture. Bake for 20 minutes. Remove from oven.

5. Carefully arrange squash, onion, and garlic evenly on sheet pan around chicken. Spread or brush all but the reserved ¼ cup honey-mustard mixture over chicken and vegetables.

6. Bake for 35 minutes or until chicken is cooked through and vegetables are tender. Brush with reserved ¼ cup honey-mustard mixture. Remove from oven and let rest for 5 to 10 minutes before serving.

Notes

____

____

____

Recipe from Julia Rutland, *Squash: 50 Tried & True Recipes*

Turkey-and-Winter Squash Pot Pie

Makes 6 servings

4 tablespoons butter

3 ribs celery, chopped

1 medium-size onion, chopped

2½ cups cubed butternut squash or pumpkin

¼ cup all-purpose flour

2 teaspoons poultry seasoning

½ teaspoon salt

1 cup chicken or turkey broth

1 cup half-and-half

3 cups chopped or shredded cooked turkey

1 (15-ounce) package store-bought refrigerated piecrusts

1 egg, lightly beaten

1. Preheat oven to 375°.

2. Melt butter in a large saucepan over medium heat. Add celery and onion. Cook, stirring frequently, for 5 minutes. Add squash. Cover and cook, stirring occasionally, for 10 minutes or until vegetables are almost tender.

3. Stir in flour, poultry seasoning, and salt. Cook for 1 minute.

4. Add broth and half-and-half, stirring until well blended. Reduce heat and simmer for 5 minutes or until thickened and bubbly. Stir in turkey.

5. Place 1 piecrust in bottom of a 9-inch pie plate. Add turkey mixture and cover with remaining crust. Fold over edges and crimp to seal. Make several slits in top. Brush with egg.

6. Bake for 30 to 40 minutes or until golden brown and bubbly.

Notes

____

____

____

____

Recipe from Julia Rutland, *Squash: 50 Tried & True Recipes*

Beef Tagine with Winter Squash

A tagine pot is a shallow, round pan with a conical lid. The design enables condensation to rise to the top, condense, then drip down to baste the food, keeping it moist and succulent. Check the manufacturer's instructions, as many clay tagines cannot be used on a cooktop. Some tagines have steel or cast-iron bases, which are safe for gas or electric cooktops.

Makes 4 servings

---

1 tablespoon paprika

2 teaspoons salt

1½ teaspoons ground cumin

½ teaspoon ground cinnamon

½ teaspoon ground ginger

½ teaspoon crushed red pepper flakes

1 teaspoon smoked paprika

1 pound lean boneless beef, cut into cubes

2 tablespoons olive oil

1 small sweet onion, chopped

2 garlic cloves, minced

1 cup beef, chicken, or vegetable broth

1 (28-ounce) can crushed or diced tomatoes, undrained

1 (1½-pound) butternut squash or pumpkin, peeled and cubed

½ cup golden raisins

Hot cooked couscous

¼ cup chopped fresh cilantro

1. Combine paprika, salt, cumin, cinnamon, ginger, pepper flakes, and paprika in a large bowl. Add beef, tossing to coat. (Beef may be refrigerated for several hours until ready to cook.)

2. Heat oil in a large (cooktop-safe) tagine bottom, Dutch oven, or soup pot over medium-high heat. Add beef and onion; cook, stirring occasionally, until beef is browned on all sides. Add garlic; cook for 1 minute.

3. Stir in broth and tomatoes; cook for 5 minutes. Add squash and raisins. Cover, reduce heat to low, and cook for 25 minutes or until squash is tender. Serve over couscous and sprinkle with cilantro.

Recipe from Julia Rutland, *Squash: 50 Tried & True Recipes*

Roasted Winter Squash, Sausage, and Brussels Sprouts

Makes 4 servings

3 cups cubed butternut squash or pumpkin

1 pound fresh Brussels sprouts, halved or quartered

12 to 16 ounces smoked sausage, sliced

⅓ cup dried cranberries

3 tablespoons extra-virgin olive oil

2 tablespoons maple syrup

1 teaspoon salt

¼ teaspoon coarsely ground black pepper

1. Preheat oven to 425°. Line a rimmed baking sheet with nonstick aluminum foil or a silicone baking mat.

2. Combine squash, sprouts, sausage, and cranberries in a large bowl. Drizzle with olive oil, maple syrup, salt, and pepper, tossing to coat.

3. Spread squash mixture in a single layer on prepared baking sheet. Bake for 30 minutes or until golden brown and tender.

4. Carefully remove from oven and drizzle with additional maple syrup. Return to oven and bake for 10 more minutes.

Notes

Recipe from Julia Rutland, *Squash: 50 Tried & True Recipes*

Winter Squash-and-Spinach Lasagna

Makes 8 servings

Vegetable cooking spray

2 (12-ounce) packages frozen butternut squash or pumpkin puree (about 2 cups), thawed

2 cups ricotta cheese, divided

¾ cup milk

1 tablespoon chopped fresh sage

2 teaspoons salt, divided

1 (10-ounce) package frozen chopped spinach, thawed and lightly squeezed dry

2 cups (8 ounces) shredded reduced-fat mozzarella cheese, divided

½ cup (2 ounces) freshly grated Parmesan cheese, divided

¼ teaspoon coarsely ground black pepper

9 no-boil lasagna noodles, divided

1. Preheat oven to 400°. Lightly grease a 13x9-inch baking dish with cooking spray.

2. Combine squash, 1 cup ricotta cheese, milk, sage, and 1½ teaspoons salt in a bowl.

3. In a separate bowl, combine spinach, remaining 1 cup ricotta, 1 cup mozzarella, ¼ cup Parmesan cheese, remaining ½ teaspoon salt, and pepper.

4. Spread ½ of squash mixture in bottom of prepared baking dish. Arrange 3 noodles over sauce (noodles will appear small but will increase in size as they cook and absorb liquid). Top with ½ of spinach mixture and 3 noodles. Repeat with remaining ½ squash mixture, remaining 3 noodles, and remaining ½ spinach mixture. Sprinkle with remaining 1 cup mozzarella and remaining ¼ cup Parmesan cheese.

5. Cover with aluminum foil and bake for 30 minutes. Uncover and bake for 15 more minutes or until lasagna is bubbly and cheese is golden brown. Let cool for 10 minutes.

Recipe from Julia Rutland, *Squash: 50 Tried & True Recipes*

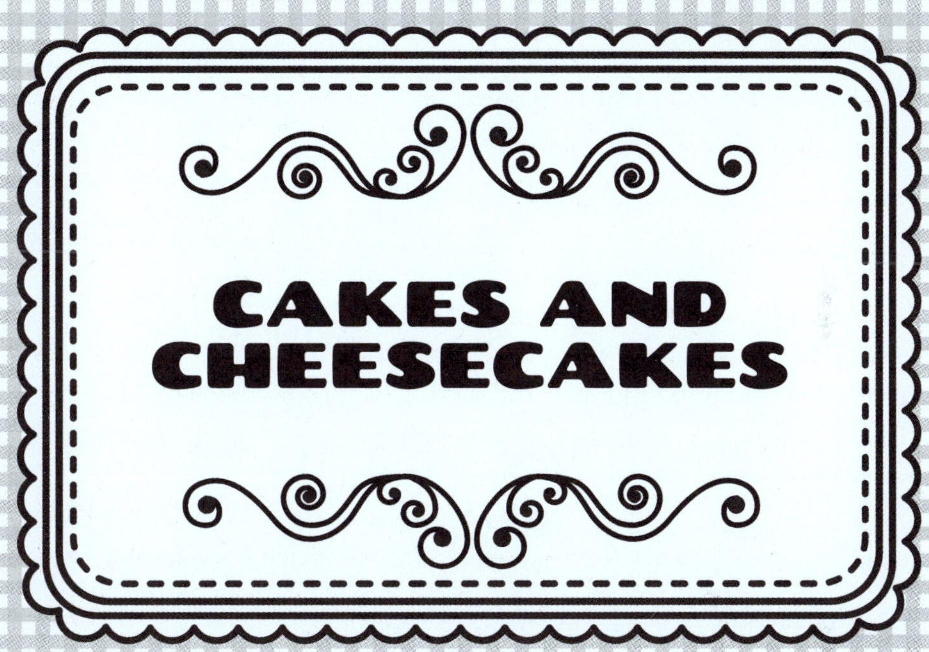
CAKES AND
CHEESECAKES

Pumpkin Sheet Cake with Cream Cheese Frosting

Makes 24 servings

---

1. Preheat oven to 350°. Lightly grease a 15x10-inch baking pan with cooking spray.

2. Beat granulated sugar, pumpkin, oil, and eggs in a large bowl.

3. In a separate bowl, combine flour, baking powder, salt, cinnamon, ginger, and cloves. Stir flour mixture into pumpkin mixture, mixing well. Pour batter into prepared pan. Bake for 20 to 25 minutes or until a wooden pick inserted in center comes out clean. Cool completely in pan on a wire rack.

4. To make frosting, beat cream cheese, butter, and vanilla in a large bowl. Gradually beat in powdered sugar until smooth. Spread over cooled cake. Store, covered, in the refrigerator.

Vegetable cooking spray

1½ cups granulated sugar

1 (15-ounce) can pumpkin (not pie mix)

1 cup vegetable oil

4 eggs

2 cups all-purpose flour

2 teaspoons baking powder

¼ teaspoon salt

2 teaspoons ground cinnamon

¼ teaspoon ground ginger

⅛ teaspoon ground cloves

1 (8-ounce) package cream cheese, softened

½ cup butter, softened

1½ teaspoons vanilla extract

5 cups powdered sugar

Notes

Recipe from Theresa Millang, *The Joy of Squash*

Choc-Dot Pumpkin Mini-Cupcakes

Makes 100 mini-cupcakes

Vegetable cooking spray

2 cups all-purpose flour

2 teaspoons baking powder

1 teaspoon baking soda

½ teaspoon salt

1½ teaspoons ground cinnamon

½ teaspoon ground cloves

¼ teaspoon allspice

¼ teaspoon ground ginger

2 cups granulated sugar

4 eggs

1 (15-ounce) can pumpkin (not pie mix)

1 cup vegetable oil

1 cup All-Bran cereal

¾ cup (6 ounces) semisweet chocolate chips

1 cup chopped nuts

2 tablespoons butter, softened

1½ cups powdered sugar

2 teaspoons lemon juice

2 tablespoons orange juice

1. Preheat oven to 350°. Lightly grease mini-cupcake pans with cooking spray.

2. Sift together flour, baking powder, baking soda, salt, cinnamon, cloves, allspice, ginger, and granulated sugar in a large bowl.

3. In a separate large bowl, beat eggs until foamy. Stir in pumpkin, oil, and cereal, mixing well. Add flour mixture to pumpkin mixture, stirring until just combined. Stir in chocolate chips and nuts. Spoon batter into prepared pans, filling ⅔ full.

4. Bake for 20 to 25 minutes. Cool.

5. To make glaze, beat together butter, powdered sugar, and juices in a small bowl until creamy. Pour over cupcakes.

Recipe from Margie Knoblauch and Mary Brubacher, *North Country Cabin Cooking*

Frosted Pumpkin Cupcakes

Makes 24 cupcakes

- 2⅓ cups all-purpose flour
- 1 teaspoon baking powder
- ½ teaspoon baking soda
- ½ teaspoon salt
- 1 tablespoon pumpkin pie spice
- ½ teaspoon ground cinnamon
- ¼ teaspoon ground nutmeg
- 2½ cups granulated sugar
- 1¼ cups butter, softened and divided
- 3 eggs
- 1 (15-ounce) can pumpkin (not pie mix)
- 2 teaspoons vanilla extract, divided
- 1 cup buttermilk
- 1 (8-ounce) package cream cheese, softened
- 4 cups powdered sugar

1. Preheat oven to 350°. Place 24 cupcake liners in 2 (12-cup) muffin pans.

2. Combine flour, baking powder, baking soda, salt, pie spice, cinnamon, and nutmeg in a large mixing bowl.

3. In the bowl of a stand-up electric mixer, beat granulated sugar and ¾ cup butter on medium speed until light and fluffy. Add eggs, 1 at a time. Beat in pumpkin and 1 teaspoon vanilla. Gradually beat in flour mixture alternately with buttermilk. Spoon batter into prepared muffin cups, filling ¾ full.

4. Bake for 20 to 25 minutes or until a wooden pick inserted in center comes out clean. Cool in pans for 10 minutes. Remove from pans. Cool completely.

5. To make frosting, beat together remaining ½ cup butter, cream cheese, remaining 1 teaspoon vanilla, and powdered sugar in a large bowl until creamy. Frost cupcakes. Store in the refrigerator.

Recipe from Theresa Millang, *The Joy of Squash*

Pumpkin Cream Cupcakes

Makes 24 cupcakes

---

1 (18.25-ounce) package spice cake mix

1 (1.34-ounce) package vanilla instant pudding mix

1 cup canned pumpkin (not pie mix)

1 (8-ounce) package cream cheese, softened

¼ cup granulated sugar

1 egg

1 teaspoon vanilla extract

1. Preheat oven to 350°. Place 24 cupcake liners in 2 (12-cup) muffin pans.

2. In a large bowl, prepare cake batter according to package directions. Stir in dry pudding mix and pumpkin, mixing well. Spoon batter into prepared muffin cups.

3. In the bowl of a stand-up electric mixer, beat cream cheese on medium speed until creamy. Beat in sugar, egg, and vanilla until well blended; spoon mixture equally over batter in muffin cups.

4. Bake for 18 to 22 minutes or until a wooden pick inserted in center comes out clean. Cool in pans for 5 minutes; remove and cool completely on a wire rack. Store in the refrigerator.

Notes

Recipe from Theresa Millang, *The Joy of Squash*

Ali's Pumpkin Crumb Cake

Makes 20 servings

1 (30-ounce) can pumpkin pie mix

1 (5-ounce) can evaporated milk

2 large eggs, lightly beaten

1 teaspoon vanilla extract

1 (18.25-ounce) package yellow cake mix

1 stick (8 tablespoons) butter, melted

½ cup chopped pecans

1. Preheat oven to 350°. Lightly grease a 13x9-inch baking pan with butter.

2. Mix together pumpkin pie mix, evaporated milk, eggs, and vanilla in a large bowl until well blended. Pour pumpkin mixture into prepared baking pan.

3. In a separate bowl, combine cake mix, melted butter, and pecans, mixing on low speed with an electric mixer until crumbly. Sprinkle crumb mixture over filling in pan.

4. Bake for 50 to 55 minutes or until top is golden brown. Remove pan from oven. Cool completely in pan on a wire rack. Cut into bars. Refrigerate leftovers.

Notes

Recipe from Theresa Millang, *The Joy of Squash*

Pumpkin-Apple Bundt Cake

Makes 12 servings

1½ cups butter, softened and divided

2 teaspoons vanilla extract, divided

2 cups powdered sugar

3½ cups all-purpose flour

1 tablespoon baking powder

2½ teaspoons ground ginger

½ teaspoon pumpkin pie spice

½ teaspoon baking soda

½ teaspoon salt

1 cup granulated sugar

½ cup light brown sugar, firmly packed

4 large eggs

1 (15-ounce) can pumpkin (not pie mix)

1 cup shredded, peeled tart apple

½ cup molasses

1. Preheat oven to 350°. Grease (with butter) and flour a 12-cup Bundt pan.

2. To make hard sauce, beat together ½ cup butter, 1 teaspoon vanilla, and powdered sugar in a medium-size bowl until fluffy. Set aside.

3. Combine flour, baking powder, ginger, pie spice, baking soda, and salt in a medium-size bowl. In the large bowl of a stand-up electric mixer, beat remaining 1 cup butter, granulated sugar, and brown sugar on low speed until creamy. Beat in eggs, 1 at a time. Beat in pumpkin, apple, molasses, and remaining 1 teaspoon vanilla. On low speed, gradually add flour mixture to pumpkin mixture. Spoon batter into prepared pan.

4. Bake for 50 to 55 minutes or until a wooden pick inserted in center comes out clean. Cool in pan on a wire rack for 15 minutes; invert onto a serving plate. Dust with powdered sugar before serving. Serve warm with reserved hard sauce. Refrigerate leftovers.

Recipe from Theresa Millang, *The Joy of Squash*

Pumpkin-Coconut Snack Cake

Makes 20 servings

1 (18.25-ounce) package yellow cake mix, divided

2 large eggs

1⅔ cups canned pumpkin pie mix

2 teaspoons pumpkin pie spice

1 teaspoon vanilla extract

½ cup flaked coconut

¼ cup chopped pecans or walnuts

3 tablespoons butter, softened

1. Preheat oven to 350°. Lightly grease a 13x9-inch baking pan with butter.

2. In a large bowl, combine 3 cups dry cake mix, eggs, pumpkin pie mix, pie spice, and vanilla; beat on low speed with an electric mixer until moistened, then beat on medium speed for 2 minutes. Pour into prepared pan.

3. In a small bowl, mix together coconut, pecans, and remaining dry cake mix. Cut in butter with a pastry blender or 2 knives until crumbly. Sprinkle coconut mixture over batter in pan.

4. Bake for 30 to 35 minutes or until a wooden pick inserted in center comes out clean. Cool in pan on a wire rack. Refrigerate leftovers.

Notes

Recipe from Theresa Millang, *The Joy of Squash*

Pumpkin Dump Cake

Makes 12 servings

All-purpose flour

1 (15-ounce) can pumpkin (not pie mix)

1 cup granulated sugar

1½ teaspoons ground cinnamon

1 teaspoon ground ginger

½ teaspoon ground cloves

½ teaspoon salt

1 (12-ounce) can evaporated milk

1 teaspoon vanilla extract

4 eggs

1 (18.25-ounce) package yellow cake mix

1 cup chopped pecans

½ cup butter, melted

1. Preheat oven to 350°. Grease (with butter) and flour a 13x9-inch baking pan.

2. In a large bowl, stir together pumpkin, sugar, cinnamon, ginger, cloves, and salt until blended. Stir in evaporated milk and vanilla. Beat in eggs, 1 at a time. Pour mixture into prepared pan.

3. Sprinkle dry cake mix over pumpkin mixture in pan; sprinkle evenly with pecans, and drizzle evenly with butter.

4. Bake for 50 to 60 minutes or until edges are lightly browned. Cool in pan on a wire rack. Serve cake warm or at room temperature. Refrigerate leftovers.

Notes

Recipe from Theresa Millang, *The Joy of Squash*

Pumpkin Pound Cake

Makes 16 servings

1. Preheat oven to 350°. Grease (with butter) and flour a 12-cup Bundt pan.

2. Combine flour, baking powder, baking soda, salt, and pie spice in a large bowl.

3. In the bowl of a stand-up mixer, beat granulated sugar and 1½ cups butter on medium speed until creamy. Beat in eggs, 1 at a time. Beat in pumpkin and 1 teaspoon vanilla. Reduce speed to low. Gradually add flour mixture to pumpkin mixture, alternately with milk, until well blended. Spoon batter into prepared pan.

4. Bake for 55 to 60 minutes or until a wooden pick inserted in center comes out clean. Cool in pan for 10 minutes. Remove from pan; cool completely.

5. To make glaze, whisk together powdered sugar, remaining 3 tablespoons butter, orange juice, and remaining ¼ teaspoon vanilla. Pour glaze over top of cake just before serving. Refrigerate leftovers.

3¾ cups all-purpose flour

1½ teaspoons baking powder

1 teaspoon baking soda

1 teaspoon salt

2 teaspoons pumpkin pie spice

2 cups granulated sugar

1½ cups (3 sticks) plus 3 tablespoons butter, softened and divided

6 eggs

¾ cup canned pumpkin (not pie mix)

1¼ teaspoons vanilla extract, divided

¾ cup whole milk

1½ cups powdered sugar

4 to 6 teaspoons fresh orange juice

Notes

Recipe from Theresa Millang, *The Joy of Squash*

Pumpkin-Pecan Dessert

Makes 16 servings

1 (15-ounce) can pumpkin (not pie mix)

¾ cup granulated sugar

¾ cup heavy cream or whole milk

3 large eggs

1 teaspoon ground cinnamon

1 teaspoon salt

1 teaspoon vanilla extract

1 (15.25-ounce) package yellow cake mix

1½ cups chopped pecans

1 cup butter, melted

Sweetened whipped cream (optional)

1. Preheat oven to 350°. Line a 13x9-inch baking pan with nonstick aluminum foil.

2. Combine pumpkin, sugar, cream, eggs, cinnamon, salt, and vanilla in a large bowl. Spoon batter into prepared pan.

3. Sprinkle cake mix evenly over top of batter in pan. Sprinkle evenly with pecans. Drizzle evenly with butter.

4. Bake for 55 to 60 minutes or until set. Cool completely; cut into squares.

5. Serve with sweetened whipped cream, if desired.

Notes

Recipe from Julia Rutland, *Squash: 50 Tried & True Recipes*

Pumpkin-Cream Cheese Roll

Makes 12 servings

Vegetable cooking spray

3 eggs

1 cup granulated sugar

⅔ cup canned pumpkin (not pie mix)

¾ cup all-purpose flour

1 teaspoon baking soda

1 teaspoon ground cinnamon

1 teaspoon ground ginger, divided

¼ teaspoon ground nutmeg

½ cup finely chopped walnuts

⅓ cup butter, softened

2 (3-ounce) packages cream cheese, softened

1 teaspoon vanilla extract

1½ cups powdered sugar

1. Preheat oven to 350°. Lightly grease a 15x10-inch rimmed baking sheet with cooking spray. Line with parchment paper; lightly grease. Place a kitchen towel on counter; sprinkle with powdered sugar.

2. In the bowl of a stand-up mixer, beat eggs on high until foamy. Beat in granulated sugar until well blended; beat in pumpkin.

3. In a separate bowl, combine flour, baking soda, cinnamon, ½ teaspoon ginger, and nutmeg; add flour mixture to pumpkin mixture, beating on low speed until blended. Stir in walnuts. Spread batter into prepared pan.

4. Bake for 14 minutes or until cake springs back when touched. Invert cake onto prepared towel. Lift off pan; peel off paper. Starting at 10-inch side, roll up cake in towel. Cool.

5. To make filling, beat butter and cream cheese in a bowl until creamy. Add vanilla, powdered sugar, and remaining ½ teaspoon ginger; beat on low speed until blended. Unroll cake and spread filling to within ½ inch of edges. Starting at 10-inch side, roll up cake. Wrap in plastic wrap. Chill. Sprinkle with powdered sugar. Cut into slices. Refrigerate leftovers.

Notes

Recipe from Theresa Millang, *The Joy of Squash*

Winter Squash Coffee Cake

Makes 10 servings

1 cup powdered sugar

1½ teaspoons vanilla extract, divided

Juice from 1 orange

1¼ cups granulated sugar, divided

¼ cup light brown sugar, firmly packed

2¼ cups all-purpose flour, divided

¼ cup quick oats

¼ cup chopped pecans

½ cup plus 3 tablespoons cold butter, cut into pieces

2½ teaspoons ground cinnamon, divided

2 eggs

1 cup cooked-and-mashed butternut squash or pumpkin

2 teaspoons baking powder

½ teaspoon salt

¼ teaspoon ground ginger

¼ teaspoon ground nutmeg

¼ teaspoon ground cloves

½ cup unsweetened applesauce

1. Preheat oven to 350°. Grease a 9-inch springform baking pan with butter.

2. To make glaze, whisk together powdered sugar and ½ teaspoon vanilla in a small bowl Stir in orange juice. Set aside.

3. To make crumb mixture, combine ¼ cup granulated sugar, brown sugar, ¼ cup flour, oats, pecans, 3 tablespoons butter, and 1 teaspoon cinnamon in a bowl; set aside.

4. In the bowl of a stand-up mixer, beat remaining ½ cup butter and remaining 1 cup granulated sugar on medium speed until light and creamy. Beat in eggs, squash, and remaining 1 teaspoon vanilla.

5. In a separate bowl, combine remaining 2 cups flour, baking powder, salt, remaining 1½ teaspoons cinnamon, ginger, nutmeg, and cloves. Beat flour mixture into squash mixture.

6. Spoon half of batter into prepared pan. Spread applesauce over batter. Top with half of reserved crumb mixture. Top with remaining half of batter, then remaining half of crumb mixture. Bake for 55 minutes. Cool in pan for 10 minutes; remove sides. Cool. Drizzle with reserved glaze.

Recipe from Theresa Millang, *The Joy of Squash*

Praline-Pumpkin Cheesecake

Makes 16 servings

1½ cups graham cracker crumbs

¼ cup granulated sugar

5 tablespoons butter, melted and cooled

1½ cups chopped pecans

1 cup light brown sugar, firmly packed and divided

2 tablespoons water

1 (8-ounce) package cream cheese, softened

1 teaspoon ground cinnamon

½ cup cornstarch

2 large eggs

1 teaspoon vanilla extract

1 (30-ounce) can pumpkin pie mix

1. Preheat oven to 350°.

2. To make crust, stir together graham cracker crumbs, granulated sugar, and butter in a small bowl; press mixture onto bottom and 1 inch up sides of a 9-inch springform baking pan.

3. To make topping, stir together pecans, ½ cup brown sugar, and 2 tablespoons water in a small bowl; reserve 1 cup topping mixture. Sprinkle remaining mixture over crust in pan.

4. To make filling, beat cream cheese, remaining ½ cup brown sugar, cinnamon, and cornstarch in a medium-size bowl with an electric mixer until creamy. Beat in eggs and vanilla until blended. Beat in pumpkin pie mix. Spoon pumpkin mixture over pecan mixture in pan.

5. Bake for 50 to 60 minutes or until center is almost set. Sprinkle with reserved 1 cup topping mixture. Bake for about 10 minutes or until center is set. Remove from oven. Run a thin knife around edge of cheesecake. Cool in pan. Chill, then remove side of pan. Store in the refrigerator.

Notes

Recipe from Theresa Millang, *The Joy of Squash*

Pumpkin Cheesecake

Makes 12 servings

1½ cups graham cracker crumbs

1 cup plus 3 tablespoons granulated sugar, divided

5 tablespoons butter, melted and cooled

3 (8-ounce) packages cream cheese, softened

3 eggs

1 cup canned pumpkin (not pie mix)

1½ teaspoons vanilla extract

1 teaspoon ground cinnamon

¼ teaspoon ground nutmeg

¼ teaspoon ground ginger

⅛ teaspoon ground cloves

Notes

____

____

____

____

____

1. Preheat oven to 350°. Grease a 9-inch springform pan with butter.

2. To make crust, mix together graham cracker crumbs, 3 tablespoons sugar, and butter in a small bowl. Press mixture onto bottom and 2 inches up sides of pan. Bake for 5 minutes. Cool on a wire rack.

3. To make filling, beat together cream cheese and remaining 1 cup granulated sugar in the bowl of a stand-up electric mixer on medium speed until smooth. Beat in eggs, 1 at a time. Beat in pumpkin, vanilla, cinnamon, nutmeg, ginger, and cloves until just blended. Pour pumpkin mixture into baked crust.

4. Bake for about 1 hour and 20 minutes or until center is almost set. Cool in pan for 10 minutes on a wire rack. Run a thin knife around edge to loosen cake from pan. Cool in pan for 1 hour on a wire rack, then immediately refrigerate and cool completely. Remove side of pan just before serving. Store in the refrigerator.

Recipe from Theresa Millang, *The Joy of Squash*

Winter Squash Cheesecake

Makes 8 servings

1 store-bought refrigerated deep-dish piecrust

1 (8-ounce) package cream cheese, softened

2 eggs

1 cup butternut squash or pumpkin puree

1 cup milk

1 cup granulated sugar

¼ teaspoon salt

½ teaspoon ground cinnamon

⅛ teaspoon ground nutmeg

⅛ teaspoon ground ginger

⅛ teaspoon allspice

1 teaspoon vanilla extract

1. Preheat oven to 350º. Line a 10-inch deep-dish pie plate with piecrust dough.

2. Beat cream cheese in a stand-up electric mixer until smooth. Beat in eggs and squash puree. Beat in milk, sugar, salt, cinnamon, nutmeg, ginger, allspice, and vanilla until well blended. Pour squash mixture into piecrust.

3. Bake for 40 to 45 minutes or until set. Cool on a wire rack. Store in the refrigerator.

Notes

Recipe from Theresa Millang, *The Joy of Squash*

Pretzel-Crusted Pumpkin Cheesecake Dessert

Makes 12 servings

1 (6-ounce) bag pretzel crisps, crushed into fine crumbs

6 tablespoons butter, melted

1 cup light brown sugar, divided

2 cups canned pumpkin (not pie mix)

2 (8-ounce) packages cream cheese

1 tablespoon vanilla extract

1¾ teaspoons ground cinnamon, divided

½ teaspoon ground cloves

½ cup heavy cream

½ cup toasted pecans, finely chopped

1. Preheat oven to 350°. Lightly grease a 13x9-inch glass baking dish with butter.

2. Mix together pretzel crumbs, butter, and 2 tablespoons brown sugar in a medium-size bowl; press mixture firmly into prepared dish. Bake for 10 minutes. Remove from oven; cool.

3. In the bowl of a stand-up electric mixer, beat pumpkin, cream cheese, ¾ cup brown sugar, vanilla, 1½ teaspoons cinnamon, and cloves until smooth and creamy. Pour mixture over completely cooled crust.

4. Beat cream and remaining 2 tablespoons brown sugar in a large bowl until stiff peaks form; drop by tablespoonfuls onto pumpkin mixture; carefully swirl the two mixtures together with a thin spatula. Sprinkle evenly with pecans. Sprinkle with remaining ¼ teaspoon cinnamon. Cover and chill for at least 8 hours before serving. Refrigerate leftovers.

Notes

____

____

____

____

____

____

Recipe from Theresa Millang, *The Joy of Squash*

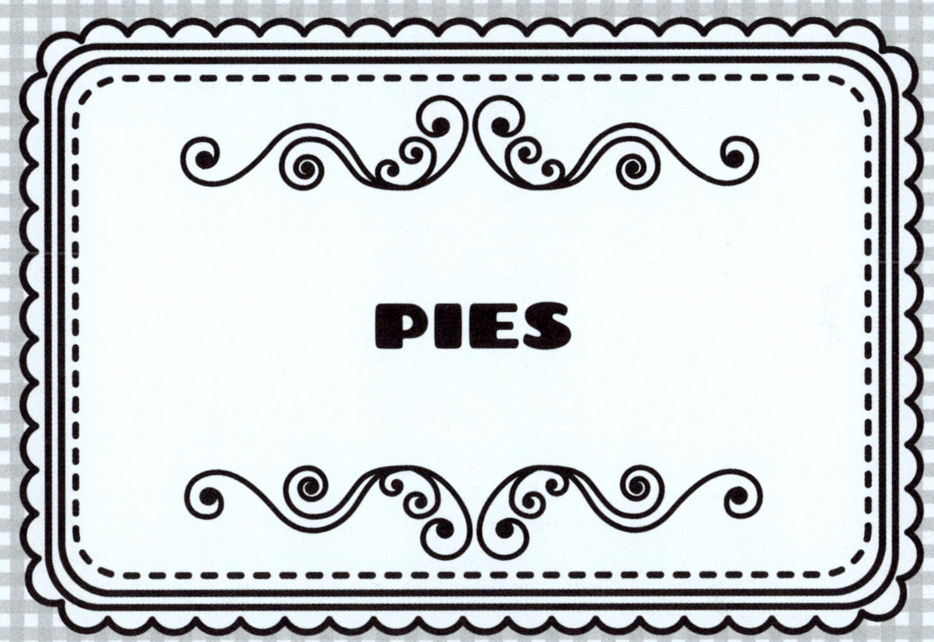

PIES

No-Crust Pumpkin Pie

Makes 1 (9-inch) pie

1. Preheat oven to 325°. Lightly grease a 9-inch pie plate with cooking spray.

2. Beat eggs in a large bowl. Add sugar, ginger, cinnamon, and salt. Stir in pumpkin. Add milk, stirring until mixture is smooth. Pour pumpkin mixture into prepared pie plate. Bake for 50 minutes or until firm or a knife inserted in filling 2 inches from center comes out clean.

Vegetable cooking spray

4 eggs

¾ cup granulated sugar

1 teaspoon ground ginger

1 teaspoon ground cinnamon

½ teaspoon salt

1 (15-ounce) can pumpkin (not pie mix)

1 cup milk

Notes

Recipe from Margie Knoblauch and Mary Brubacher, *North Country Cabin Cooking*

Spiced Pumpkin Pie

Makes 8 servings

1 store-bought refrigerated deep-dish piecrust

½ cup granulated sugar

⅓ cup light brown sugar, firmly packed

1½ teaspoons ground cinnamon

½ teaspoon salt

¾ teaspoon ground ginger

¼ teaspoon ground cloves

¼ teaspoon ground nutmeg

4 large eggs, divided

1 (15-ounce) can pumpkin (not pie mix) or 2 cups pumpkin puree

1 cup heavy cream, half-and-half, or milk

1 teaspoon vanilla extract

1. Preheat oven to 375°. Fit piecrust into a 10-inch pie plate.

2. Whisk together sugars, cinnamon, salt, ginger, cloves, and nutmeg in a small bowl.

3. Beat 3 eggs in a large bowl. Stir in pumpkin and sugar mixture. Whisk in cream and vanilla.

4. Pour mixture into piecrust. Crimp edges or decorate with additional pastry crust pieces. Lightly beat remaining egg in a small bowl; brush edges of crust with beaten egg.

5. Place pie on a baking sheet. Bake for 40 to 50 minutes, shielding crust with aluminum foil, if necessary, to prevent overbrowning. (It's okay if the pie is slightly jiggly in the center; it should firm as it cools.) To test for doneness, insert a knife near the center to see if it comes out clean. Cool on a wire rack. Serve at room temperature or chill until serving.

Notes

Recipe from Julia Rutland, *Squash: 50 Tried & True Recipes*

Creamy Two-Layer Pumpkin Pie

Makes 8 servings

2 (8-ounce) packages cream cheese, softened

½ cup granulated sugar

2 eggs

1 teaspoon vanilla extract

½ cup canned pumpkin (not pie mix)

½ teaspoon ground cinnamon

¼ teaspoon ground nutmeg

⅛ teaspoon ground cloves

1 (6-ounce) store-bought graham cracker piecrust

Notes

1. Preheat oven to 325°.

2. In the bowl of a stand-up electric mixer, beat cream cheese and sugar until smooth. Beat in eggs and vanilla. Remove 1 cup batter and place in a separate bowl; stir in pumpkin, cinnamon, nutmeg, and cloves. Pour remaining plain batter into piecrust. Top evenly with pumpkin batter.

3. Bake for about 40 minutes or until center is almost set. Cool slightly on a wire rack, then refrigerate immediately. Chill for at least 3 hours before serving. Refrigerate leftovers.

Recipe from Theresa Millang, *The Joy of Squash*

Fresh Sugar Pumpkin Pie

Makes 8 servings

1 store-bought refrigerated deep-dish piecrust

2 cups cooked, mashed sugar pumpkin

¾ cup granulated sugar

¼ teaspoon salt

1¼ teaspoons ground cinnamon

1 teaspoon ground ginger

½ teaspoon ground nutmeg

¼ teaspoon ground cloves

3 large eggs

1 (12-ounce) can evaporated milk

½ cup whole milk

1 teaspoon vanilla extract

1. Preheat oven to 400°. Line a 10-inch deep-dish pie pan with unbaked crust; flute edges.

2. Combine pumpkin, sugar, salt, cinnamon, ginger, nutmeg, and cloves in a large bowl.

3. In a separate bowl, beat eggs lightly. Add evaporated milk, whole milk, and vanilla; beat until blended. Add milk mixture to pumpkin mixture, blending well. Pour batter into unbaked piecrust until almost full (be careful not to overfill; discard any extra).

4. Bake for 50 to 60 minutes or until a knife inserted in center comes out clean. Cool completely on a wire rack. Chill before serving. Store in the refrigerator.

Notes

____

____

____

____

____

____

Recipe from Theresa Millang, *The Joy of Squash*

Apple-and-Fresh Pumpkin Pie

Makes 8 servings

- ⅓ cup light brown sugar, firmly packed
- 1 tablespoon cornstarch
- 1 teaspoon ground cinnamon, divided
- ½ teaspoon salt, divided
- ⅓ cup cold water
- 2 tablespoons butter
- 3 cups thinly sliced Granny Smith apples
- 1 (9-inch) store-bought unbaked piecrust (in pie pan)
- 1 egg
- ⅓ cup granulated sugar
- ¾ cup freshly cooked pumpkin puree
- ¼ teaspoon ground cloves
- ¼ teaspoon ground ginger
- ¾ cup evaporated milk
- 1 teaspoon vanilla extract

1. Preheat oven to 425°.

2. Combine brown sugar, cornstarch, ½ teaspoon ground cinnamon, ¼ teaspoon salt, ⅓ cup water, and butter in a medium-size saucepan. Cook over medium heat, stirring constantly, until mixture comes to a boil. Add apples, tossing to coat; cook for 4 minutes. Pour apple mixture into piecrust.

3. In a large bowl, whisk together egg, granulated sugar, pumpkin, remaining ½ teaspoon cinnamon, remaining ¼ teaspoon salt, cloves, ginger, milk, and vanilla. Spoon pumpkin mixture over apple mixture in piecrust. Bake for 10 minutes, then reduce heat to 375°. Bake for about 40 minutes or until filling is just set in the middle. Cool completely in pan on a wire rack. Refrigerate leftovers.

Recipe from Theresa Millang, *The Joy of Squash*

Pumpkin Chiffon Pie

Makes 8 servings

- 1¾ cups finely ground gingersnap cookie crumbs
- 2 tablespoons granulated sugar
- ⅓ cup melted butter
- 2 envelopes unflavored gelatin
- ¼ cup boiling water
- 1 (5-ounce) can evaporated milk
- 1 (30-ounce) can pumpkin pie mix
- 1 teaspoon vanilla extract
- 1 (3-ounce) box vanilla instant pudding and pie filling mix
- 1 teaspoon pumpkin pie spice
- 1½ cups frozen-and-thawed nondairy whipped topping

1. Preheat oven to 350°. Lightly grease a deep-dish pie plate with butter.

2. To make crust, combine cookie crumbs, sugar, and butter in a small bowl; remove ⅓ cup crumb mixture and set aside. Press remaining crumb mixture on bottom and up sides of prepared pie plate. Bake for 8 minutes. Remove from oven; cool completely on a wire rack.

3. To make filling, place gelatin in a small saucepan. Pour ¼ cup boiling water over gelatin; let stand for 1 minute. Heat gelatin over low heat until dissolved. Add evaporated milk and cook, stirring constantly, until just hot but not boiling. Remove from heat.

4. In the bowl of a stand-up electric mixer, beat pumpkin, vanilla, pudding mix, pie spice, and gelatin mixture on high speed for 3 minutes. Gently fold in whipped topping. Spoon pumpkin mixture into prepared crust. Sprinkle with ⅓ cup reserved crumb mixture. Refrigerate immediately. Chill for 2 hours or until firm enough to cut. Refrigerate leftovers.

Notes

____

____

____

____

Recipe from Theresa Millang, *The Joy of Squash*

Pumpkin-Cream Cheese Pie

Makes 8 servings

- 1 (9-inch) store-bought refrigerated piecrust
- 1 (8-ounce) package plus 1 (3-ounce) package cream cheese, softened
- 1 cup granulated sugar
- 3 tablespoons all-purpose flour
- 1½ teaspoons pumpkin pie spice
- 3 eggs
- 1 teaspoon vanilla extract
- 1 (15-ounce) can pumpkin (not pie mix)

1. Preheat oven to 375°. Fit piecrust into a 9-inch glass pie plate, following package instructions for a single-crust filled pie. Bake for about 8 minutes or until light brown. Remove from oven; set aside.

2. In a large mixing bowl, beat cream cheese and sugar with an electric mixer until smooth. Add flour, pie spice, eggs, vanilla, and pumpkin; beat until blended. Pour pumpkin mixture into prepared crust.

3. Bake for 35 to 45 minutes or until a knife inserted in center comes out clean. Cool for 30 minutes, then cover and refrigerate. Chill for 2 hours before serving. Store in the refrigerator.

Notes

Recipe from Theresa Millang, *The Joy of Squash*

Pumpkin Cream Pie

Makes 8 servings

---

1 (9-inch) store-bought refrigerated piecrust

⅓ cup plus 2 tablespoons granulated sugar, divided

1 (8-ounce) package cream cheese, softened

1½ teaspoons vanilla extract, divided

¼ teaspoon ground cardamom

3 eggs, divided

¾ cup light brown sugar, firmly packed

1 (15-ounce) can pumpkin (not pie mix)

1 tablespoon all-purpose flour

1½ teaspoons pumpkin pie spice

½ cup half-and-half

1 cup heavy cream

1. Preheat oven to 375°. Fit piecrust into a 9-inch glass pie plate, following package instructions for a single-crust filled pie. Bake for about 8 minutes or until light brown. Remove from oven; set aside.

2. Beat ⅓ cup granulated sugar, cream cheese, 1 teaspoon vanilla, and cardamom in a medium-size bowl on medium speed until fluffy. Beat in 1 egg. Spread cream cheese mixture into prepared crust.

3. In a large bowl, stir together brown sugar, remaining 2 eggs, pumpkin, flour, and pie spice until blended. Gradually stir in half-and-half. Spoon pumpkin mixture carefully over cream cheese mixture in crust. Cover edges of crust with strips of aluminum foil. Bake for 30 minutes. Remove foil; bake for 30 to 40 minutes or until a knife inserted in center comes out clean. Cool on a wire rack for 2 hours, then refrigerate.

4. To make topping, beat cream, remaining 2 tablespoons sugar, and remaining ½ teaspoon vanilla in a medium-size bowl on high speed until stiff peaks form. Spread whipped cream on chilled pie. Refrigerate leftovers.

Notes

____

____

____

Recipe from Theresa Millang, *The Joy of Squash*

Pumpkin Ice-cream Pie

Makes 8 servings

1½ cups graham cracker crumbs

3 tablespoons granulated sugar

6 tablespoons butter, melted and cooled

1 cup canned pumpkin (not pie mix)

½ cup light brown sugar, firmly packed

½ teaspoon salt

½ teaspoon ground ginger

½ teaspoon ground cinnamon

½ teaspoon ground nutmeg

1 quart vanilla ice cream

¼ cup toasted pecans, finely chopped

1. Lightly grease a 9-inch deep-dish pie plate with butter.

2. To make crust, combine graham cracker crumbs, granulated sugar, and butter in a small bowl, mixing until well blended. Press crumb mixture onto bottom of prepared pie plate. Freeze.

3. Stir together pumpkin, brown sugar, salt, ginger, cinnamon, and nutmeg in a small bowl.

4. In a large bowl, gently stir ice cream to soften, then quickly fold in pumpkin mixture until blended. Pour ice-cream mixture into prepared crust. Sprinkle pecans in a circle around outer edge of pie. Freeze until firm. Cover with aluminum foil when frozen and return to freezer. Remove from freezer 10 minutes before serving. Freeze leftovers.

Notes

Recipe from Theresa Millang, *The Joy of Squash*

Tofu-Pumpkin-Pecan Pie

Makes 12 servings

1¼ cups all-purpose flour

¼ cup pecan pieces

1 teaspoon salt, divided

½ cup plus 1 tablespoon granulated sugar, divided

½ cup vegetable shortening

2 to 3 tablespoons ice water

¾ cup pecan halves

6 tablespoons maple syrup, divided

1 (16-ounce) package extra-firm silken tofu, drained

1 (15-ounce) can pumpkin (not pie mix)

1 teaspoon vanilla extract

1 teaspoon ground cinnamon

½ teaspoon ground ginger

¼ teaspoon ground cloves

1. To make crust, place flour, pecan pieces, ½ teaspoon salt, and 1 tablespoon sugar in a food processor; pulse until pecans are finely ground. Add shortening; pulse until almost combined. Add 2 tablespoons ice water; pulse until just blended. Form dough into a ball, then press into a flat disk and wrap in plastic wrap; chill.

2. Take dough out and let stand for 15 minutes. Roll dough out onto a lightly floured surface into an 11-inch circle; fit into a 9-inch pie plate; crimp edges. Stir together pecan halves and 2 tablespoons maple syrup in a bowl, tossing to coat. Place coated pecans in bottom of piecrust.

3. Preheat oven to 400°.

4. Place tofu in a food processor; process until smooth. Add pumpkin, remaining ½ cup sugar, remaining 4 tablespoons maple syrup, vanilla, remaining ½ teaspoon salt, cinnamon, ginger, and cloves; puree until smooth. Pour pumpkin mixture into piecrust.

5. Bake for about 1 hour or until a knife inserted in center comes out clean. Cool on a wire rack. Refrigerate leftovers.

Recipe from Theresa Millang, *The Joy of Squash*

Turtle Pumpkin Pie

Makes 10 servings

¼ cup plus 2 tablespoons caramel ice-cream topping, divided

1 (6-ounce) store-bought graham cracker piecrust

½ cup plus 2 tablespoons chopped toasted pecans, divided

1 cup cold whole milk

2 (3.4-ounce) packages vanilla instant pudding mix

1 cup canned pumpkin (not pie mix)

1 teaspoon ground cinnamon

½ teaspoon ground nutmeg

⅛ teaspoon ground ginger

1 teaspoon vanilla extract

1 (8-ounce) container frozen nondairy whipped topping, thawed and divided

1. Pour ¼ cup caramel topping into piecrust, then sprinkle with ½ cup pecans.

2. Beat milk, pudding mix, pumpkin, cinnamon, nutmeg, ginger, and vanilla in a large bowl on low speed until blended. Stir in 1½ cups whipped topping. Spoon pumpkin mixture into piecrust and refrigerate immediately. Chill for 1 hour before serving.

3. Top pie with remaining ½ cup whipped topping, remaining 2 tablespoons caramel topping, and remaining 2 tablespoons pecans before serving. Store in the refrigerator.

Recipe from Theresa Millang, *The Joy of Squash*

Pumpkin Tart with Currant Glaze

Makes 1 pie (6 to 8 servings)

All-purpose flour

1 (9-inch) store-bought refrigerated piecrust

1 (15-ounce) can pumpkin

1 (8-ounce) package cream cheese, softened

2 large eggs

¾ cup granulated sugar

1 teaspoon vanilla extract or rum extract (optional)

1 teaspoon ground cinnamon

½ teaspoon ground ginger

¼ teaspoon allspice

3 cups currant juice or other dark juice

2 tablespoons cornstarch

2 tablespoons cold water

1. Position oven rack in bottom third of oven. Preheat oven to 375°. On a lightly floured surface, roll out pastry and fit into an 11-inch tart pan; trim edges slightly higher than rim of pan. Line crust with aluminum foil, pressing into corners; fill with dried beans or pie weights. Bake for 10 minutes. Remove foil and beans, then return to oven and bake for 5 to 10 minutes or until golden brown. Remove from oven.

2. Reduce oven temperature to 350°. To make filling, combine pumpkin and cream cheese in a large bowl. Beat with an electric mixer until smooth. Beat in eggs; sugar; vanilla, if desired; cinnamon; ginger; and allspice until smooth. Pour pumpkin mixture into prepared crust, smoothing top. Bake for 45 to 60 minutes or until set. Remove from oven and let cool.

3. To make glaze, boil currant juice until reduced to 2 cups. Stir cornstarch into 2 tablespoons water; add to juice in pan. Cook, stirring constantly, until thickened and bubbly. Remove from heat; cool slightly. Pour cooled juice mixture over tart, spreading and smoothing with back of spoon. Store in the refrigerator.

Notes

Recipe from Teresa Marrone, *Abundantly Wild*

Pumpkin Crisp

Makes 18 servings

1 (18.25-ounce) package yellow cake mix, divided

1 cup butter, softened and divided

3 eggs, divided

1 (29-ounce) can pumpkin (not pie mix)

1 teaspoon ground cinnamon

½ teaspoon ground nutmeg

¼ teaspoon ground ginger

1 cup granulated sugar, divided

⅔ cup evaporated milk

1 teaspoon vanilla extract

1. Preheat oven to 350°. Lightly grease a 13x9-inch baking pan with butter.

2. Remove 1 cup cake mix and set aside. Melt ½ cup butter in a medium-size bowl. Stir in remaining cake mix and 1 egg, mixing until crumbly. Pat crust mixture into prepared pan.

3. In a large bowl, combine remaining 2 eggs, pumpkin, cinnamon, nutmeg, ginger, ½ cup sugar, milk, and vanilla; pour pumpkin mixture over crust mixture in pan.

4. In a medium-size bowl, stir together reserved 1 cup cake mix, remaining ½ cup granulated sugar, and remaining ½ cup butter until coarse crumbs form; sprinkle evenly over pumpkin mixture.

5. Bake for 55 to 60 minutes. Serve warm. Refrigerate leftovers.

Notes

Recipe from Theresa Millang, *The Joy of Squash*

Mary's Little Pumpkin Pies

Makes 12 servings

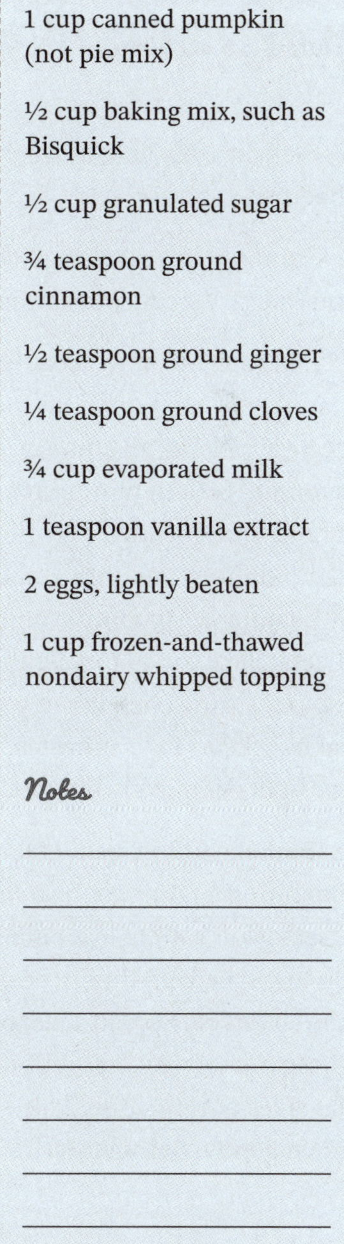

Vegetable cooking spray

1 cup canned pumpkin (not pie mix)

½ cup baking mix, such as Bisquick

½ cup granulated sugar

¾ teaspoon ground cinnamon

½ teaspoon ground ginger

¼ teaspoon ground cloves

¾ cup evaporated milk

1 teaspoon vanilla extract

2 eggs, lightly beaten

1 cup frozen-and-thawed nondairy whipped topping

Notes

1. Preheat oven to 375°. Lightly grease 1 (12-cup) muffin pan with cooking spray.

2. Combine pumpkin, baking mix, sugar, cinnamon, ginger, cloves, milk, vanilla, and eggs in a large bowl, stirring until well blended. Spoon ¼ cup mixture into each muffin cup.

3. Bake for about 30 minutes or until edges start pulling away from sides of cups. Remove from oven; cool for 10 minutes, then loosen sides of pies with a thin knife. Remove pies from cups; place on a wire rack. Cool slightly before serving. Top each pie with 1 tablespoon whipped topping. Refrigerate leftovers.

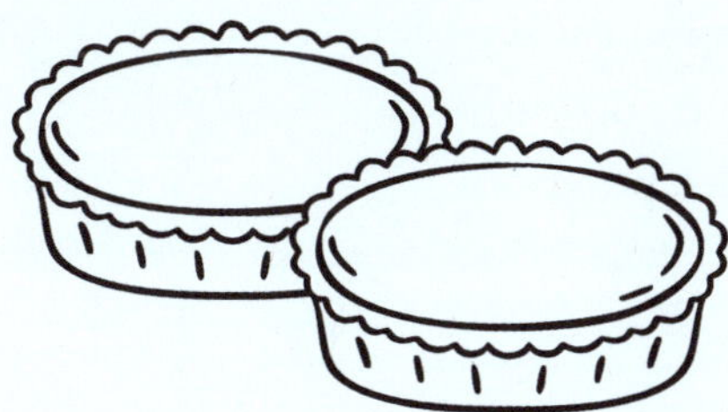

Recipe from Theresa Millang, *The Joy of Squash*

Mini-Whoopie Pumpkin Pies

Makes 36 servings

2 cups all-purpose flour

1 teaspoon baking powder

1 teaspoon baking soda

1 teaspoon ground cinnamon

½ teaspoon ground ginger

½ teaspoon salt

½ cup plus 6 tablespoons butter, softened and divided

1¼ cups granulated sugar

2 large eggs

1 cup canned pumpkin (not pie mix)

1½ teaspoons vanilla extract, divided

4 ounces cream cheese, softened

1½ cups powdered sugar

1. Preheat oven to 350°. Lightly grease 4 baking sheets with butter.

2. Combine flour, baking powder, baking soda, cinnamon, ginger, and salt in a large bowl.

3. In a separate bowl, beat ½ cup butter and granulated sugar on medium speed with an electric mixer until smooth. Beat in eggs, 1 at a time. Beat in pumpkin and 1 teaspoon vanilla until blended. Stir flour mixture into pumpkin mixture until combined. Drop dough by heaping teaspoonfuls onto prepared baking sheets. Bake for 10 to 12 minutes or until cookies spring back when touched. Cool on baking sheets for 5 minutes. Remove cookies and cool completely on wire racks.

4. To make filling, beat cream cheese, remaining 6 tablespoons butter, and remaining ½ teaspoon vanilla in a small bowl until fluffy. On low speed, gradually beat in powdered sugar until blended. Spread 1 heaping teaspoonful filling onto flat side of half of cookies. Top with flat sides of remaining half of cookies; press down gently. Refrigerate.

Notes

Recipe from Theresa Millang, *The Joy of Squash*

Cake Mix-Pumpkin Pie Dessert

Makes 15 servings

1 (18.25-ounce) package spice cake mix, divided

¾ cup butter, softened and divided

3 large eggs, divided

⅔ cup whole milk

1 (30-ounce) can pumpkin pie mix

1 teaspoon vanilla extract

¼ cup light brown sugar, firmly packed

½ cup chopped pecans

1. Preheat oven to 350°. Lightly grease a 13x9-inch baking pan with butter.

2. Remove 1 cup cake mix and set aside. Melt ½ cup butter.

3. To make crust, beat together melted butter, remaining cake mix, and 1 egg in a large bowl with an electric mixer on low speed until well blended. Spread batter in bottom of prepared baking pan.

4. In same bowl, beat remaining 2 eggs, milk, pumpkin, and vanilla until smooth; pour pumpkin mixture over crust mixture in pan.

5. In a medium-size bowl, mix reserved 1 cup cake mix, brown sugar, and remaining ¼ cup butter until coarse crumbs form. Stir in pecans; sprinkle over pumpkin mixture.

6. Bake for 50 to 60 minutes or until a knife inserted in center comes out clean. Cool in pan for 15 minutes. Cut into squares. Serve warm or cool. Store in the refrigerator.

Notes

Recipe from Theresa Millang, *The Joy of Squash*

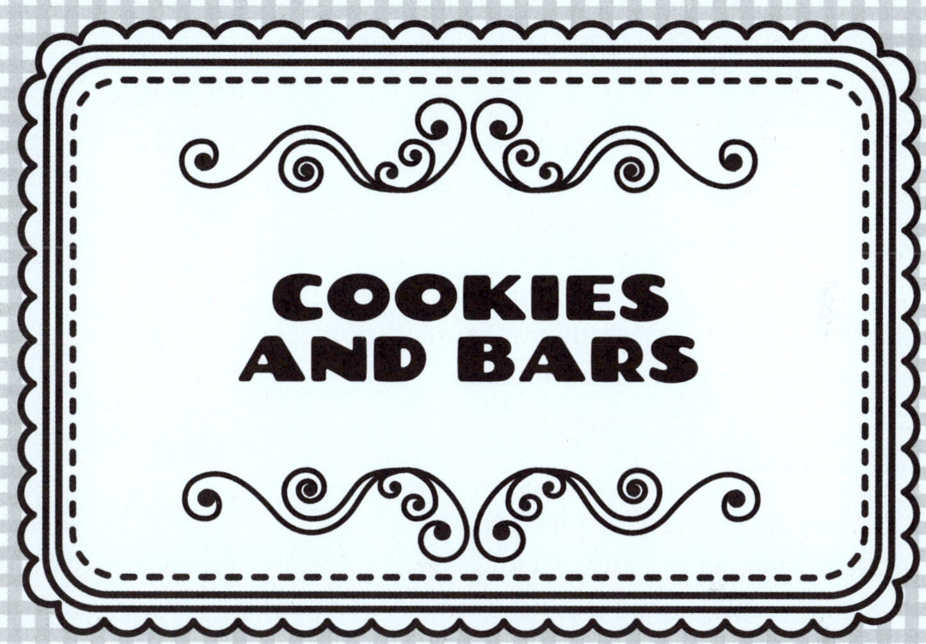

COOKIES AND BARS

Mitzi's Golden Pumpkin Cookies

Makes 4 dozen cookies

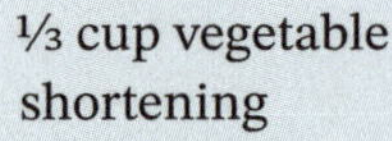

⅓ cup vegetable shortening

1⅓ cups granulated sugar

3 eggs, well beaten

1 cup canned pumpkin (not pie mix)

1 teaspoon vanilla extract

1 teaspoon lemon extract

1 teaspoon grated lemon rind

¼ teaspoon allspice

1 teaspoon ground cinnamon

¼ teaspoon ground ginger

1 teaspoon ground nutmeg

2½ cups all-purpose flour

4 teaspoons baking powder

1 teaspoon salt

1 cup raisins

1. Preheat oven to 400°. Lightly grease a baking sheet with shortening.

2. Cream shortening and sugar in a large bowl. Add eggs, pumpkin, vanilla, and lemon extract.

3. In a separate bowl, combine lemon rind, allspice, cinnamon, ginger, nutmeg, flour, baking powder, and salt. Stir flour mixture into pumpkin mixture until a soft dough forms. Dredge raisins in a little flour; mix coated raisins into dough.

4. Drop dough by tablespoonfuls onto prepared baking sheet. Sprinkle with sugar and cinnamon. Bake for 15 minutes.

Notes

Recipe from Mary Ann Winkowski, *Beyond Delicious*

Cream Cheese-Frosted Walnut-Pumpkin Cookies

Makes 5 dozen cookies

1¼ cups butter, softened and divided

⅔ cup light brown sugar, firmly packed

⅓ cup granulated sugar

1 cup canned pumpkin (not pie mix)

1 egg

2 teaspoons vanilla extract, divided

2 cups all-purpose flour

1½ teaspoons pumpkin pie spice

1 teaspoon baking powder

1 teaspoon baking soda

¼ teaspoon salt

1 cup chopped walnuts

2 cups powdered sugar

1 (3-ounce) package cream cheese, softened

1. Preheat oven to 350°.

2. In the bowl of a stand-up electric mixer, beat 1 cup butter, brown sugar, and granulated sugar on medium speed until creamy. Add pumpkin, egg, and 1 teaspoon vanilla; beat until blended.

3. Reduce speed to low; add flour, pie spice, baking powder, baking soda, and salt. Beat until well blended. Stir in walnuts.

4. Drop dough by rounded teaspoonfuls, 2 inches apart, onto ungreased baking sheets. Bake for 8 to 10 minutes or until set. Cool completely.

5. To make frosting, beat powdered sugar, remaining ¼ cup butter, cream cheese, and remaining 1 teaspoon vanilla in a medium-size bowl until smooth; cover and store in the refrigerator. Frost cookies just before serving. Refrigerate leftovers.

Notes

Recipe from Theresa Millang, *The Joy of Squash*

Oatmeal-Raisin-Pumpkin Cookies

Makes 4 dozen cookies

- 2 cups all-purpose flour
- 1⅓ cups quick oats
- 1 teaspoon baking soda
- 1 teaspoon ground cinnamon
- ½ teaspoon salt
- 1 cup butter, softened
- 1 cup light brown sugar, firmly packed
- 1 cup granulated sugar
- 1 cup canned pumpkin (not pie mix)
- 1 large egg
- 1 teaspoon vanilla extract
- ¾ cup coarsely chopped walnuts
- ¾ cup raisins

1. Preheat oven to 350°. Lightly grease baking sheets with butter.

2. Combine flour, oats, baking soda, cinnamon, and salt in a large bowl; set aside.

3. In the bowl of a stand-up electric mixer, beat butter, brown sugar, and granulated sugar on medium speed until light and fluffy. Beat in pumpkin, egg, and vanilla.

4. Reduce speed to low and gradually add flour mixture to pumpkin mixture, beating until well blended. Stir in chopped walnuts and raisins. Drop by rounded tablespoonfuls onto prepared baking sheets.

5. Bake for 14 to 16 minutes or until lightly browned and set in centers. Cool on baking sheets for 2 minutes, then remove and cool completely on wire racks. Refrigerate leftovers.

Notes

____

____

____

____

____

Recipe from Theresa Millang, *The Joy of Squash*

Pumpkin Cheesecake Cups

Makes 12 servings

1. Preheat oven to 325°. Place 12 cupcake liners in a muffin pan.

2. Mix together cookie crumbs and butter in a small bowl. Press equal amounts onto the bottom of each muffin cup. Bake for 4 minutes. Remove from oven.

3. In the bowl of a stand-up electric mixer, beat cream cheese and sugar until creamy. Add pumpkin, pie spice, and vanilla; beat until blended. Add eggs; beat well. Spoon batter equally into cups, filling ¾ full.

4. Bake for 25 to 30 minutes. Cool in pan on a wire rack. Remove cups from pan and refrigerate. Serve chilled. Refrigerate leftovers.

⅔ cup crushed gingersnaps

2 tablespoons butter, melted and cooled

1 (8-ounce) package cream cheese, softened

½ cup granulated sugar

1 cup canned pumpkin (not pie mix)

1 teaspoon pumpkin pie spice

1 teaspoon vanilla extract

2 large eggs

Notes

Recipe from Theresa Millang, *The Joy of Squash*

Pumpkin Bars

Makes 3 dozen

2 cups all-purpose flour

2 teaspoons baking powder

1 teaspoon baking soda

½ teaspoon salt

2 teaspoons ground cinnamon

2 cups granulated sugar

4 eggs, beaten

1 (15-ounce) can pumpkin (not pie mix)

1 cup vegetable oil

3 ounces cream cheese, softened

6 tablespoons butter

1 teaspoon milk

1 teaspoon vanilla extract

1¾ cups powdered sugar

1. Preheat oven to 350°.

2. Combine flour, baking powder, baking soda, salt, cinnamon, and granulated sugar in a large bowl. Add eggs, pumpkin, and oil, mixing well. Spread pumpkin mixture onto a rimmed baking sheet; bake for 25 minutes.

3. To make frosting, stir together cream cheese, butter, milk, vanilla, and powdered sugar in a large bowl. Spread on cooled cake. Cut into bars.

Notes

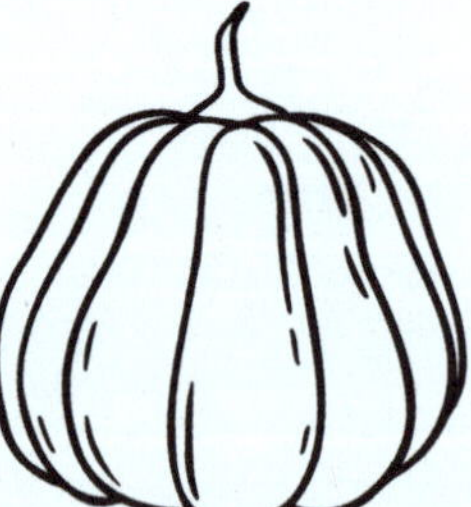

Recipe from Margie Knoblauch and Mary Brubacher, *North Country Cabin Cooking*

Cream Cheese-Pumpkin Bars

Makes 49 bars

- 4 eggs
- 2 cups granulated sugar
- 1 cup vegetable oil
- 1 (15-ounce) can pumpkin (not pie mix)
- 2 teaspoons vanilla extract, divided
- 2 cups all-purpose flour
- 2 teaspoons baking powder
- 1 teaspoon baking soda
- ¼ teaspoon salt
- 2 teaspoons ground cinnamon
- ½ teaspoon ground ginger
- ¼ teaspoon ground cloves
- 1 cup dark raisins
- 1 (8-ounce) package cream cheese, softened
- ¼ cup butter, softened
- 2 to 3 tablespoons milk
- 4 cups powdered sugar
- ½ cup finely chopped walnuts (optional)

1. Preheat oven to 350°. Lightly grease a 15x10-inch baking pan with butter.

2. In a large bowl, beat eggs, granulated sugar, oil, pumpkin, and 1 teaspoon vanilla extract until smooth.

3. In a separate bowl, combine flour, baking powder, baking soda, salt, cinnamon, ginger, and cloves. Stir flour mixture into pumpkin mixture. Stir in raisins. Spread batter into prepared pan. Bake for 25 to 30 minutes or until a wooden pick inserted in center comes out clean. Cool completely in pan on a wire rack.

4. To make frosting, beat cream cheese, butter, milk, and remaining 1 teaspoon vanilla with an electric mixer in a medium-size bowl until smooth. On low speed, gradually beat in powdered sugar, 1 cup at a time, until smooth. Spread over cold bars; sprinkle with nuts, if desired. Cut 7 rows long by 7 rows wide. Store in the refrigerator.

Recipe from Theresa Millang, *The Joy of Squash*

Winter Squash Cheesecake Bars

Makes 18 bars

- ½ cup old-fashioned oats
- 10 full-size graham crackers
- ½ cup plus 2 tablespoons granulated sugar, divided
- ¼ cup plus 3 tablespoons all-purpose flour, divided
- 2 tablespoons butter
- 3 tablespoons milk
- 2 (8-ounce) packages reduced-fat cream cheese, softened
- 2 large eggs
- ½ cup butternut squash or pumpkin puree
- 1 teaspoon vanilla extract
- ½ teaspoon ground cinnamon
- ¼ teaspoon ground nutmeg
- ¼ teaspoon salt

1. Preheat oven to 350°. Lightly grease a 13x9-inch baking pan with butter.

2. To make crust, place oats, graham crackers, 2 tablespoons sugar, ¼ cup flour, and butter in a food processor; process until finely ground. Add milk; pulse to moisten. Pat mixture into bottom of prepared pan. Bake for 10 minutes. Cool on a wire rack.

3. Reduce heat to 325°. In the bowl of a stand-up electric mixer, beat cream cheese and remaining ½ cup sugar on medium speed until creamy. Beat in eggs, 1 at a time. Beat in squash puree, vanilla, cinnamon, nutmeg, salt, and remaining 3 tablespoons flour. Spread squash mixture over prepared crust.

4. Bake for about 35 minutes or until set. Cool completely in pan on a wire rack, then immediately refrigerate. Chill before cutting into bars. Store in the refrigerator.

Notes

Recipe from Theresa Millang, *The Joy of Squash*

Frosted Pumpkin Bars

Makes 60 bars

1½ cups all-purpose flour

1¼ cups granulated sugar

2 teaspoons baking powder

1 teaspoon baking soda

¼ teaspoon salt

2 teaspoons ground cinnamon

½ teaspoon ground ginger

1¼ cups butter, melted, cooled, and divided

1 (15-ounce) can pumpkin (not pie mix)

3 eggs, lightly beaten

1½ teaspoons vanilla extract, divided

¾ cup dried sweetened cranberries, chopped

4 cups powdered sugar

¼ cup orange juice

1. Preheat oven to 350°.

2. Combine flour, sugar, baking powder, baking soda, salt, cinnamon, and ginger in a large bowl. Add ¾ cup butter, pumpkin, eggs, ½ teaspoon vanilla, and cranberries, stirring until well blended. Spread batter into an ungreased rimmed baking sheet. Bake for 20 to 25 minutes or until a wooden pick inserted in center comes out clean. Cool completely in pan on a wire rack.

3. To make frosting, mix remaining ½ cup butter, powdered sugar, and remaining 1 teaspoon vanilla in a medium-size bowl. Stir in just enough orange juice to reach a desired spreading consistency. Frost cooled bars. Cut and serve. Refrigerate leftovers.

Notes

____

____

____

Recipe from Theresa Millang, *The Joy of Squash*

Pecan Pie-Pumpkin Bars

Makes 12 bars

1 cup all-purpose flour

½ cup quick oats

¾ cup light brown sugar, firmly packed and divided

½ cup butter, softened

¾ cup granulated sugar

1 (15-ounce) can pumpkin (not pie mix)

1 (12-ounce) can evaporated milk

2 eggs

2 teaspoons pumpkin pie spice

1 teaspoon vanilla extract

½ cup chopped pecans

Whipped cream

1. Preheat oven to 350°.

2. Combine flour, oats, ½ cup brown sugar, and butter in a bowl; beat with an electric mixer on low speed until crumbly. Press flour mixture into a 13x9-inch baking pan. Bake for 15 minutes.

3. In the bowl of a stand-up electric mixer, beat granulated sugar, pumpkin, evaporated milk, eggs, pie spice, and vanilla on medium speed for 2 minutes; pour pumpkin mixture over prepared crust. Bake for 20 minutes.

4. Stir together pecans and remaining ¼ cup brown sugar in a small bowl. Sprinkle pecan mixture over top. Bake for 15 to 25 minutes or until a knife inserted in center comes out clean. Cool completely in pan on a wire rack. Cut into bars. Serve topped with whipped cream. Refrigerate leftovers.

Notes

____

____

____

____

____

____

____

Recipe from Theresa Millang, *The Joy of Squash*

Ice-cream Pumpkin Squares

Makes 9 servings

1¼ cups graham cracker crumbs

¼ cup butter, softened

1 tablespoon granulated sugar

1 cup canned pumpkin (not pie mix)

½ cup light brown sugar, firmly packed

½ teaspoon ground cinnamon

½ teaspoon ground ginger

¼ teaspoon ground nutmeg

1 quart vanilla ice cream (4 cups), softened

1. To make crust, mix together graham cracker crumbs, butter, and granulated sugar in a small bowl; press crumb mixture evenly and firmly onto bottom of a 9-inch-square baking pan.

2. Combine pumpkin, brown sugar, cinnamon, ginger, and nutmeg in a large bowl. Stir in softened ice cream with a spoon; spread over crust in pan. Freeze, uncovered, until firm. Cover and store in the freezer. When ready to serve, remove from freezer 10 minutes before cutting into squares. Freeze leftovers.

Notes

Recipe from Theresa Millang, *The Joy of Squash*

Pumpkin Pie Squares

Makes 15 servings

1 cup all-purpose flour

½ cup quick oats

½ cup light brown sugar, firmly packed

1 stick butter, softened

1 (15-ounce) can pumpkin (not pie mix)

1 (13½-ounce) can evaporated milk

2 eggs

¼ cup granulated sugar

½ teaspoon salt

½ teaspoon ground cinnamon

½ teaspoon ground ginger

½ teaspoon ground cloves

1. Preheat oven to 350°. Lightly grease a 9x13-inch baking pan with butter.

2. To make crust, combine flour, oats, brown sugar, and butter until crumbly. Press crust mixture flat into prepared pan. Bake for 15 minutes. Let cool.

3. To make filling, whisk together pumpkin, evaporated milk, eggs, granulated sugar, salt, cinnamon, ginger, and cloves in a large bowl. Pour pumpkin mixture over cooled crust. Bake for 20 minutes or until center is set and no longer wobbly. Let cool completely and cut into bars. Store in the refrigerator.

Notes

____

____

____

____

____

____

Recipe from Holly Harden, *Recipes for Gatherings from Mrs. Sundberg's Kitchen*

Spicy Pumpkin Dessert Squares

Makes 15 servings

1½ cups light brown sugar, firmly packed and divided

¼ cup granulated sugar

1 (29-ounce) can pumpkin (not pie mix)

1 (12-ounce) can evaporated milk

5 eggs

1 teaspoon vanilla extract

2 teaspoons ground cinnamon

½ teaspoon ground ginger

½ teaspoon ground cloves

¾ cup all-purpose flour

¼ cup cold butter, cut into small pieces

½ cup chopped pecans

1. Preheat oven to 350°. Lightly grease a 13x9-inch baking dish with butter.

2. In a large bowl, beat together 1 cup brown sugar, granulated sugar, pumpkin, evaporated milk, eggs, vanilla, cinnamon, ginger, and cloves until smooth. Pour pumpkin mixture into prepared baking dish. Bake for 20 to 25 minutes or until partially set.

3. In a small bowl, mix flour, remaining ½ cup brown sugar, and butter with a pastry blender or fork until coarse crumbs form. Stir in pecans. Sprinkle nut mixture over hot, partially baked pumpkin mixture, and bake for 15 to 20 minutes or until a knife inserted in center comes out clean. Cool in baking dish for 30 minutes, then refrigerate and cool completely. Cut into squares. Store in the refrigerator.

Notes

Recipe from Theresa Millang, *The Joy of Squash*

Date-and-Pecan Pumpkin Squares

Makes 24 squares

2½ cups whole wheat pastry flour

1½ teaspoons baking powder

¾ teaspoon ground cinnamon

½ teaspoon ground nutmeg

½ teaspoon ground cloves

½ teaspoon salt

1 cup plus 2 tablespoons butter, softened

1 cup light brown sugar, firmly packed

2 large eggs

1 cup canned pumpkin (not pie mix)

1 teaspoon vanilla extract

¼ cup cold water

3 cups pitted dates, roughly chopped

1 cup toasted chopped pecans

1. Preheat oven to 350°. Lightly grease a 13x9-inch baking pan with butter.

2. Combine flour, baking powder, cinnamon, nutmeg, cloves, and salt in a large bowl.

3. In a separate bowl, beat butter and brown sugar with an electric mixer. Beat in eggs, 1 at a time. Add pumpkin, vanilla, and ¼ cup water; beat until well blended. Mix dates with ¼ cup flour mixture in a small bowl. Gradually add remaining flour mixture to pumpkin mixture. Stir in floured dates and pecans. Spread batter into prepared baking pan.

4. Bake for about 1 hour or until a wooden pick insert in center comes out clean. Cool in pan on a wire rack. Cut into squares. Store in the refrigerator.

Recipe from Theresa Millang, *The Joy of Squash*

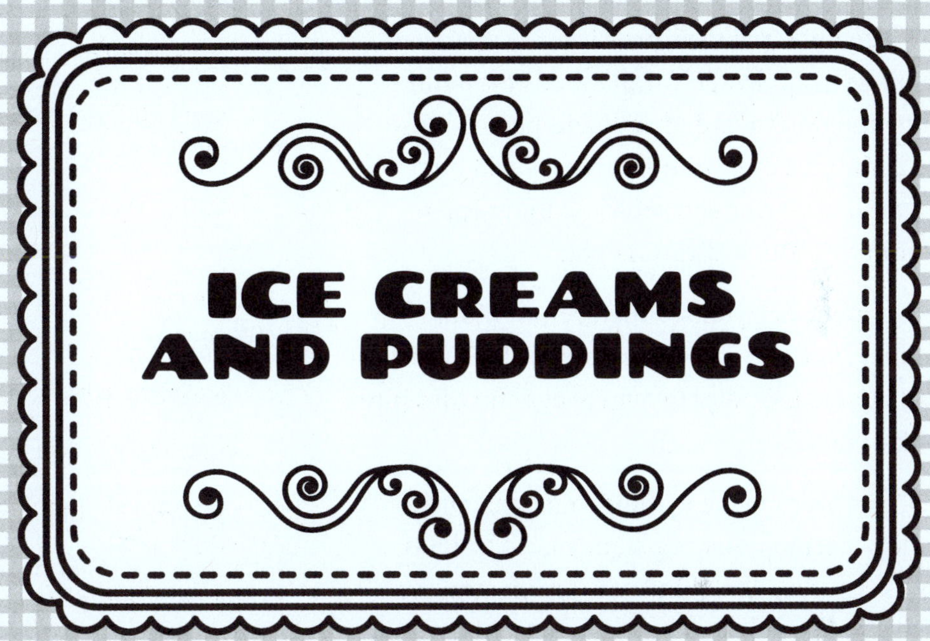

ICE CREAMS AND PUDDINGS

Pumpkin Spice Ice Cream

Makes about 8 cups

2 cups milk

1 vanilla bean, split lengthwise

8 egg yolks

¾ cup granulated sugar

¼ cup light brown sugar, firmly packed

1½ teaspoons ground cinnamon

½ teaspoon ground nutmeg

½ teaspoon salt

3 cups heavy cream

1 cup canned pumpkin (not pie mix)

Spiced or toasted pecans (optional)

1. Place milk in a medium-size saucepan over medium heat. Scrape vanilla seeds into milk, whisking until blended, and add pod. Cook for 2 minutes or until mixture is warm but not boiling. Cover and set aside for at least 30 minutes. Discard vanilla pod.

2. Combine egg yolks, sugars, cinnamon, nutmeg, and salt in a large bowl. Whisk until well blended. Gradually whisk egg mixture into milk mixture.

3. Cook over low heat, whisking constantly, until a thermometer registers 160°. Strain, if necessary, through a fine wire-mesh strainer to remove any cooked egg pieces. Cool to room temperature.

4. Combine egg mixture, cream, and pumpkin. Cover and chill until cold. (For best flavor, allow mixture to chill overnight.)

5. Pour pumpkin mixture into the freezer container of an ice-cream maker. Freeze according to manufacturer's instructions. Pack into a plastic food container; cover and freeze until firm. Serve with pecans, if desired.

Notes

Recipe from Julia Rutland, *Squash: 50 Tried & True Recipes*

Pumpkin-Cookie Ice Cream

Makes 8 servings

1 pint heavy cream

½ cup whole milk

1 cup light brown sugar, firmly packed

1 cup canned pumpkin (not pie mix)

1 teaspoon ground cinnamon

¾ teaspoon ground ginger

¼ teaspoon salt

2 teaspoons vanilla extract

½ cup coarsely broken gingersnaps

1. In a large bowl, combine cream, milk, brown sugar, pumpkin, cinnamon, ginger, salt, and vanilla. Strain mixture into an ice-cream maker; freeze following manufacturer's instructions.

2. Place ice cream in a medium-size bowl; stir in gingersnaps. Spoon mixture into a clean plastic food container; cover and freeze for about 3 hours or until ready to serve. Store, covered, in the freezer. Makes about 1 quart.

Notes

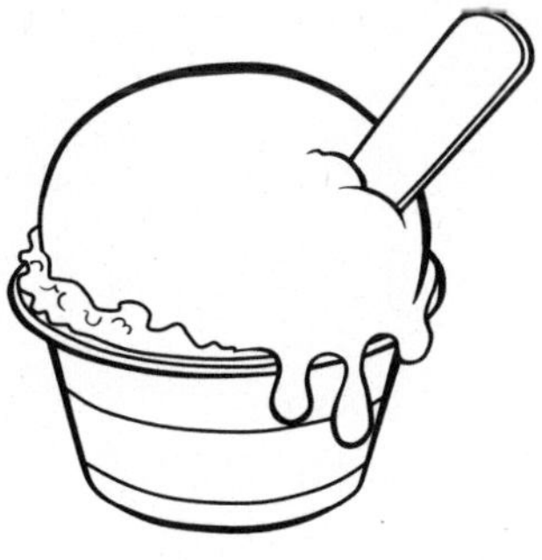

Recipe from Theresa Millang, *The Joy of Squash*

Pumpkin-Cream Cheese Parfaits

Makes 6 servings

1 (8-ounce) package cream cheese or Neufchâtel

1 cup canned pumpkin (not pie mix)

5 tablespoons maple syrup, divided

6 tablespoons honey

¾ teaspoon ground cinnamon, divided

⅛ teaspoon ground nutmeg

1 cup heavy cream

½ teaspoon vanilla extract

½ cup chopped pecans, divided

1. Beat cream cheese in a medium-size bowl until smooth. Add pumpkin, 3 tablespoons maple syrup, honey, ½ teaspoon cinnamon, and nutmeg; beat on low speed until blended.

2. Beat cream with an electric mixer in a medium-size bowl until soft peaks form. Add vanilla, remaining 2 tablespoons maple syrup, and remaining ¼ teaspoon cinnamon; beat until stiff peaks form.

3. Spoon half of pumpkin mixture evenly into 6 parfait glasses. Top evenly with half of whipped cream and ¼ cup pecans. Repeat layers with remaining half of pumpkin mixture, remaining half of whipped cream, and remaining ¼ cup pecans. Chill. Serve. Refrigerate leftovers.

Notes

Recipe from Theresa Millang, *The Joy of Squash*

No-Cook Pumpkin Pudding

Makes 4 servings

1½ cups cold whole milk

1 cup heavy cream, divided

1 (3.4-ounce) package vanilla instant pudding mix

¾ teaspoon ground cinnamon

¼ teaspoon ground ginger

¼ teaspoon ground cloves

1 cup canned pumpkin (not pie mix)

1 teaspoon vanilla extract, divided

1 tablespoon granulated sugar

1. In a medium-size bowl, whisk together milk, ½ cup cream, pudding mix, cinnamon, ginger, and cloves for about 3 minutes or until thickened and smooth. Add pumpkin and ½ teaspoon vanilla, stirring until blended. Spoon pudding into 4 dessert dishes.

2. In a small bowl, whip remaining ½ cup cream, remaining ½ teaspoon vanilla, and sugar until stiff peaks form. Spoon equal dollops onto each serving. Serve or refrigerate immediately. Refrigerate leftovers.

Notes

Recipe from Theresa Millang, *The Joy of Squash*

Country Pumpkin Custard

Makes 4 servings

1 (15-ounce) can pumpkin (not pie mix)

2 eggs, lightly beaten

1 cup half-and-half

1 teaspoon vanilla extract

⅔ cup plus ¼ cup light brown sugar, firmly packed and divided

1½ teaspoons pumpkin pie spice

½ teaspoon salt

¼ cup chopped pecans

1 tablespoon butter, melted

1. Preheat oven to 350°. Lightly grease 4 (10-ounce) custard baking cups with butter.

2. Combine pumpkin, eggs, half-and-half, vanilla, ⅔ cup brown sugar, pie spice, and salt, stirring until well blended. Pour pumpkin mixture equally into prepared baking cups. Place cups in a 13x9-inch baking pan; pour hot water around cups to a depth of 1 inch. Bake for 20 minutes.

3. In a small bowl, mix together remaining ¼ cup brown sugar, pecans, and melted butter. Sprinkle nut mixture equally over filling in cups and bake for about 35 minutes or until a knife inserted in center comes out clean. Cool slightly on a wire rack. Serve warm or cool. Store in the refrigerator.

Notes

Recipe from Theresa Millang, *The Joy of Squash*

Pumpkin Bread Pudding

Makes 15 servings

- 5 cups freshly cooked pumpkin puree
- 2 whole eggs plus 2 egg yolks
- 3 cups half-and-half
- 1 teaspoon vanilla extract
- ¼ cup dark brown sugar, firmly packed
- 1¼ cups granulated sugar, divided
- ¾ teaspoon ground cinnamon
- ¼ teaspoon ground nutmeg
- ¼ teaspoon ground cardamom (optional)
- 2 tablespoons cold water
- 1 cup heavy cream, divided
- 10 cups (2-inch) cubes challah bread or Italian bread, divided

Notes

____

____

____

1. In a large bowl, combine pumpkin; whole eggs; egg yolks; half-and-half; vanilla; brown sugar; ¼ cup granulated sugar; cinnamon; nutmeg; and, if desired, ground cardamom. Set pumpkin mixture aside.

2. In a small saucepan, mix 2 tablespoons cold water and remaining 1 cup granulated sugar. Heat over high heat. As sugar melts, swirl pan often for even melting (do not stir with a spoon). Cook for about 3 to 4 minutes or until sugar has a deep caramel color. Remove from heat.

3. Carefully whisk ¼ cup cream into caramel until combined, then whisk in remaining ¾ cup cream. Pour cream mixture into a 2½-quart baking dish. Top with half of bread cubes, then pour half of reserved pumpkin mixture over top. Top with remaining half of bread cubes, then with remaining half of pumpkin mixture. Let sit for 30 minutes.

4. Preheat oven to 350°.

5. Bake for about 35 to 45 minutes or until set. Serve. Refrigerate leftovers.

Recipe from Theresa Millang, *The Joy of Squash*

Substitutions

BAKING POWDER	
1 teaspoon	¼ teaspoon baking soda + ½ teaspoon cream of tartar
BISCUIT MIX	
1 cup	1 cup all-purpose flour + 1½ teaspoons baking powder + 2 tablespoons shortening or butter
BREADCRUMBS	
1 cup	¾ cup cracker crumbs
BROTH	
1 cup	1 cup boiling water + 1 bouillon cube or 1 teaspoon granules or paste
BUTTERMILK	
1 cup	1 cup milk + 1 tablespoon lemon juice or vinegar
1 cup	1 cup plain yogurt
CHOCOLATE	
1 ounce unsweetened	3 tablespoons cocoa powder + 1 tablespoon butter or vegetable oil
1 ounce unsweetened	1½ ounces semisweet and remove 1 tablespoon sugar from recipe
1 ounce bittersweet or semisweet	⅔ ounce unsweetened chocolate + 2 teaspoons sugar
1 ounce bittersweet	1 ounce semisweet
1 ounce semisweet	1 ounce unsweetened + 1 tablespoon sugar
1 ounce sweet baking chocolate	3 tablespoons cocoa powder + 4 teaspoons sugar + 1 tablespoon butter or vegetable oil
CORN SYRUP (LIGHT)	
1 cup	¾ cup sugar + ¼ cup additional liquid in recipe
CORN SYRUP (DARK)	
1 cup	¾ cup light corn syrup + ¼ cup molasses

FLOUR, ALL-PURPOSE FLOUR (FOR THICKENING)	
2 tablespoons	1 tablespoon cornstarch
2 tablespoons	2 tablespoons quick-cooking tapioca
FLOUR, CAKE	
1 cup	1 cup - 2 tablespoons all-purpose + 2 tablespoons cornstarch
FLOUR, SELF-RISING	
1 cup	1 cup all-purpose + 1½ teaspoons baking powder + ⅛ teaspoon salt
HALF-AND-HALF	
1 cup	½ cup milk + ½ cup whipping cream
HERBS	
1 tablespoon fresh	1 teaspoon dried
LEMON JUICE	
1 teaspoon fresh juice	½ teaspoon vinegar
MOLASSES	
1 cup	1 cup almond butter
PEANUT BUTTER	
1 cup	1 cup almond butter
SUGAR (LIGHT BROWN)	
1 cup	½ cup dark brown sugar + ½ cup granulated sugar
SUGAR (GRANULATED)	
1 cup	1¾ cups powdered
1 cup	1 cup firmly packed light brown sugar
TOMATO SAUCE	
2 cups	1 cup tomato paste + 1 cup water

Sources

Harden, Holly. *Recipes for Gatherings from Mrs. Sundberg's Kitchen.* Adventure Publications, 2015.

Knoblauch, Margie and Mary Brubacher. *North Country Cabin Cooking.* Adventure Publications, 2019.

Kozlak, Corrine. *Maple Syrup: 40 Tried & True Recipes.* Adventure Publications, 2020.

Lund, Dr. Duane R. *Cooking Minnesotan You-Betcha!: Recipes from the Kitchens of Minnesota.* Adventure Publications, 2001.

Lund, Dr. Duane R. *The Soup Cookbook: More than 150 Soup, Stew and Chili Recipes!* Adventure Publications, 1999.

Marrone, Teresa. *Abundantly Wild: Collecting and Cooking Wild Edibles in the Upper Midwest.* Adventure Publications, 2004.

Marrone, Teresa. *The Seasonal Cabin Cookbook.* Adventure Publications, 2001.

Millang, Theresa. *The Joy of Squash: From Acorn to Zucchini.* Adventure Publications, 2013.

Rutland, Julia. *Cast-Iron Cooking.* Adventure Publications, 2025.

Rutland, Julia. *Squash: 50 Tried & True Recipes.* Adventure Publications, 2019.

Winkowski, Mary Ann. *Beyond Delicious.* Clerisy Press, 2025.

Index

N

P

Q

R

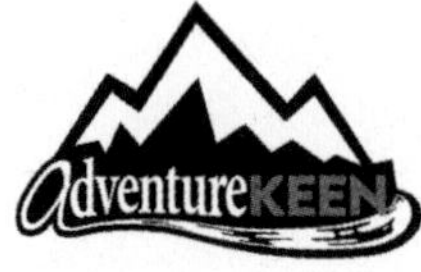

The Story of AdventureKEEN

We are an independent nature and outdoor activity publisher. Our founding dates back more than 40 years, guided then and now by our love of being in the woods and on the water, by our passion for reading and books, and by the sense of wonder and discovery made possible by spending time recreating outdoors in beautiful places.

It is our mission to share that wonder and fun with our readers, especially with those who haven't yet experienced all the physical and mental health benefits that nature and outdoor activity can bring.

In addition, we strive to teach about responsible recreation so that the natural resources and habitats we cherish and rely upon will be available for future generations.

We are a small team deeply rooted in the places where we live and work. We have been shaped by our communities of origin—primarily Birmingham, Alabama; Cincinnati, Ohio; and the northern suburbs of Minneapolis, Minnesota. Drawing on the decades of experience of our staff and our awareness of the industry, the marketplace, and the world at large, we have shaped a unique vision and mission for a company that serves our readers and authors.

We hope to meet you out on the trail someday.

#bewellbeoutdoors